Weight Loss Starts in Your Brain

Veronique Cardon, M.S.

Weight Loss Starts in Your Brain
by Veronique Cardon, M.S.

Published by
The CogniDiet®
Princeton, NJ
www.TheCogniDiet.com

ISBN: 978-0-692-98883-1

Printed in the United States

Cover design and layout by Eric Labacz, www.labaczdesign.com

CogniDiet® Table of Contents

Introduction

People always ask me what is different about The CogniDiet®. The answer is that contrary to a typical diet, we focus the teaching and support on self-discovery and personal transformation. "Weight loss starts in your brain®." This is where all decisions start: The behaviors, the habits, the addictions, and the thoughts have been ingrained there for years. When you start a diet you just think about calories, points, restrictions, and allowed foods you may not really like. Let's be honest; you are not really happy. The result is you can't wait to go back to your old habits. And so after a while the old habits, and the weight, come back with a vengeance. The CogniDiet® uses cognitive behavior therapy, brain neuroplasticity, and stress relief techniques to guide you toward long term change and results. Your brain is plastic which means no matter your age, it remains flexible and adaptable. It also means it can learn new things.

The success of our 12-week program—or just six weeks for some participants—over the past three years, as well as our clinical trial in 2016, inspired me to write a book so that I could help people outside the Princeton, NJ, area. Our work has proved that steady will win the race. We confirmed it in a clinical trial with 40 women aged 41 to 74 who lost an average of 12 pounds (a maximum of 33 pounds). We also demonstrated they lowered their total cholesterol, LDL, and triglycerides. The book's 12-week curriculum follows The CogniDiet® plan so that you can work it on your own or share it with friends and family. There is a group discussion guide after each chapter and we also offer a webinar series that can guide you specifically through the program, week after week.

We have created eye-opening tips, mind shifts, self-discovery games, and experiments to help you transform. It's one thing to say you want to lose the weight, but then you must take action! By playing with these experiments you will learn new things and adopt new behaviors. This book guides you holistically to a lifestyle free from dependency on certain foods.

The secret is that you have to be ready to change. You must want something different than the usual diet. You must be willing to jump off the never-ending dieting merry-go-round. You must want to free yourself. If you are the person who:

✓ **Has been yoyo dieting all her life**
✓ **Has tried every diet possible, miracle supplement, milk shake, special food, medication, and possibly deprivation**
✓ **Is worried about the impact of weight on her health**
✓ **Knows she is out of tricks and needs to change her lifestyle**
✓ **Is open to learn and go on a path of self-discovery**

Then you are perfect for this program and you will succeed, my friend. I did, and have been at my healthy weight since 2005. Enjoy the journey, take your time, discover a few things about yourself and lose weight naturally.

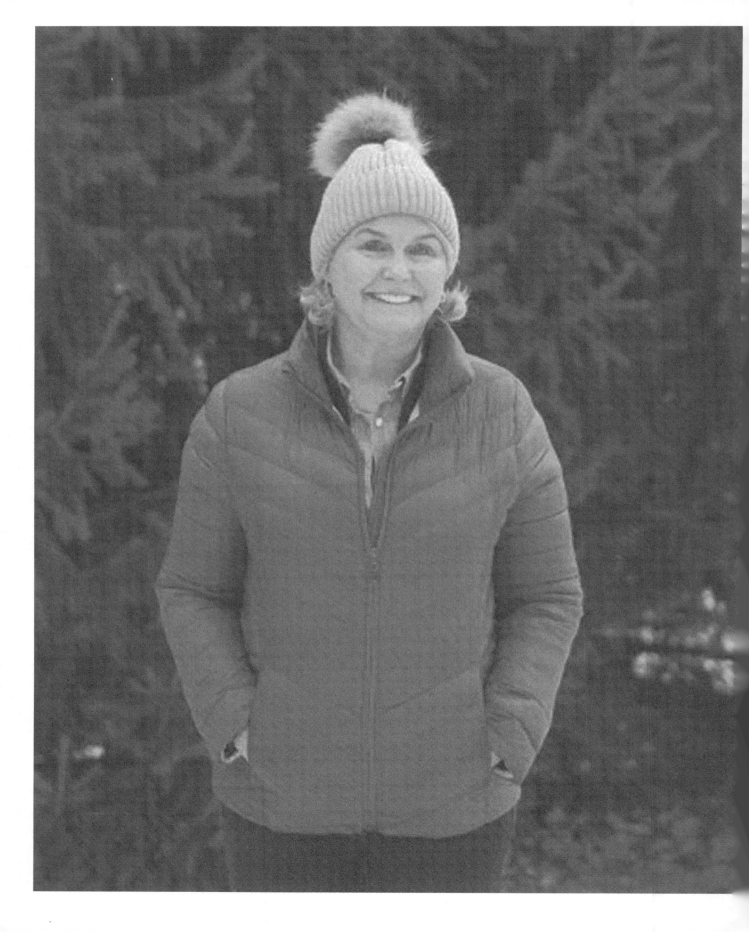

My Story

You Can Choose to Live a Healthier Life and Be Happy

Yes, this is a book about weight loss. But before we embark on this journey together, I want you to know me better and understand my story; it has shaped the creation of this program.

When Disease Hits

Cancer should have been my wake-up call. But when you live a miracle, you start to believe you are invincible. This is what happened to me. I was diagnosed with ovarian cancer in 2001; they caught the tumor quickly, and when my surgeon, Dr. Goldberg, woke me up, I saw great relief in his eyes. I knew I was safe. He told me I would not need chemotherapy or radiation because the cancerous cells were contained.

Everything was gone, the ovaries and the uterus. Bye bye maternity.

The signs of disease had been accumulating. I experienced haphazard monthly bleeding patterns, and my belly started to grow as if I was pregnant. I felt tired all the time and lost weight. The irony of it was that when I started to inexplicably lose weight, all the alarm bells went off. The sad part of the story is I had been working in the pharmaceutical and health industry for 20 years. I should have known better. But I never put myself first. I thought good health and longevity, which run in my family, were bestowed upon me like a sure gift.

I, like most of us, had a powerful ability to convince myself there was no problem; that the issue would just go away. I would be young forever. I acted as if a magic wand waved above my belly could make everything all right. My ability for denial was unlimited.

This is the story of a very successful business woman, blessed with great health, who did not listen to her body, heart or mind; who did not pay attention to how she fed herself, and who did not accept she had limits. The 30-pound weight gain was a metaphor: I covered up the issues with a few layers of extra fat.

After this miraculous intervention, and with a new spring in my step, I started an amazing, yet even more stressful job which required extensive commuting to New York in August 2001. You would think I would have known better.

Now multiply the stress triggering factors. Add a high responsibility and pressure job to a longer commute, to late nights, to no time to enjoy life, and you have a catastrophe in the making. I remember that all I was doing during weekends was sleep. And when up, I was eating sugar and sweets mindlessly, to soothe the pain. What was I thinking?

Puffy, Overeating and Tired

A few years later, in 2004, I was a sorry vision of what I used to be. I should have taken better care of myself. I was overweight, puffy, always tired. Health indexes such as cholesterol and blood sugar were elevated. I even managed to have a fatty liver at what—45? I had become a stress eater, grabbing any chocolate or crappy cookie I could find after a tough meeting. I sadly had adopted the American diet and had discovered fried foods, Cherry Coke®, and hamburgers while living my first years in the U.S., and guess where, in Atlanta. The land of fried everything! I went from being a rather skinny European with healthy habits to a fast food eater. I lost my roots. I did not pay attention to food portions. I did not pay attention to all the sugar hidden in everything. I drank gigantic milkshakes.

Combine this with stress, and you get a catastrophic weight gain. I remember scouting the empty office space at 7 p.m. with an uncontrollable craving for anything sugary. It did not solve any problem. It did not really make me feel better, only puffier, more tired, and more bloated. It's as if I had abandoned my body and self-esteem. There was no nourishment of the soul or the body. I had fat rolls everywhere. Even the appearance of my fat had changed. There was no discipline in eating, no rules. Bear claws were my best friend, even one hour before dinner, on my way back home. I became a constant muncher. I was not exercising. I remember licking ice cream on the train coming back from New York City at 6 p.m. I entered a vicious circle of not feeding my body right, which in turn diminished my energy, intellectual acuity, sex drive and self-esteem. Sugar became my drug.

Hello Depression!

And then it happened. The second message from the universe hit me. In 2005 I experienced, at the office, in the middle of a meeting, what would be my first panic attack.

If you ever had a panic attack, think back to it. You believe you are dying of a heart attack or a stroke. You don't know what hits you. For me, it started in my feet with a tingling that went up my body like a tsunami to finally hit the heart hard. It felt like a huge wave of negative electric energy traversing my body, leaving me completely disoriented. I remember hiding in a room and walking nonsensically about to try to calm down. I must have looked like a fly trapped in a glass. I tried to escape and there was no way out. A panic attack is the ultimate symptom of a person not able to fight or flee. Paralyzed with fear.

But there is a way out. I had to find the courage to go to the exit. I knew that, but I was not ready to face it. I had to realize first that I had not allowed myself to be a priority in my own life. I was smart enough to recognize the pattern of a panic attack. I did my homework. But I also started to act very strangely, hiding in the bathroom each time I thought one was coming at the office. I vividly remember being seated on the loo, crying, feeling lost and lonely. This sense of being totally alone in the world is the most painful emotion I remember experiencing at that time. But I talked to nobody, including my family. This was my secret shame. I was very good at pretending. Ovarian cancer was something I was comfortable explaining to people around me. We found a solution, I got surgery, and it got cured. I had not needed chemotherapy; I didn't live through that agony and physical pain. I did not carry that stigma. Maybe this is why I brushed it off so easily. But panic attacks are a condition you hide. You feel diminished, you believe you are weak, you think you are a loser. As an executive in a field dominated by men, I felt I was not possessing the steely resolve and self-control my profession required. I managed a lot of people. I could not show weakness. I was presenting a good front—for a while. But I felt like a failure inside.

After a while, my family and friends noticed I was withdrawn and sad. I was not fun to be around. I look at old pictures of myself at that time and do not recognize myself. I started to realize that I was maybe not cut out for the corporate world, but I was the bread winner and I had two young girls. So I plowed ahead. I was courageously going toward what I knew had a bad ending. But I did not allow myself to come first. Better to eat a 600-calorie coffee and cupcake than face your issues. This sugar roller-coaster also influenced my ability to be focused and heal my brain.

I ask myself now, why did I let myself get to the end of the rope? There is this human deeply ingrained belief that our bodies will carry us forever. Somebody said once, "Our body would die for us." Sure, especially, if we do not feed it well.

I had to take a medical leave from my job twice. Once for three months at the end of 2005, and again in the spring of 2006 because I came back too early the first time. The panic attacks were becoming more frequent and more violent. I had a hard time focusing, making decisions, and my thoughts were not clear. I knew my work was impacted. I was exhausted all the time. I was diagnosed with severe anxiety and depression, but what is called a high-functioning depression. I was not suicidal, I was just brain dead. In a strange twist, because it created more stress, at the end of 2005 I enrolled in an online nutrition class to gain a master's degree. I was following my survival instincts; realizing I needed a better understanding of how food and nutrients could help me feel better. And why the heck I was always turning to sugar. I knew I had to care for and love my neglected body. I craved a body, mind and career change.

Stress Broke My Brain

I saw a psychiatrist who told me I had broken my brain because of stress. I had allowed myself to be at my highest level of stress for too long. You will learn in this book that it is very important to recognize and address your stress level. And you will also learn that too much stress can make you fat! Because, as we will see later, excessive stress causes elevated levels of the hormone cortisol that has been shown to contribute to abdominal obesity or "belly fat." I could not write, read, drive or even cook. I was at home, like a wilted flower, watching TV on the sofa, out of any ounce of energy. Everything was too much for me. We adopted a young dog who died on Valentine's Day. I cried for days. I could not watch a sad movie, I could not watch the news. Any small decision was too much for me to make and threw me into a panic.

This created tension in the family as I was the decision maker. I was emotionally detached from my kids and husband, uninterested in any social life. I took Lexapro®, Wellbutrin® and Klonopin® when a panic attack was coming. In May 2006, I slowly started to feel better. I was finally letting my deepest feelings out. I recognized my heart was bleeding. Everything had been bottled up for too long. I had buried, deep inside, many unresolved issues from my youth. I took care of them with food. I swallowed my pain with a chocolate cookie. I realized, with the help of a wonderful psycho-therapist, that my whole career obsession was based on an unmet need to impress my father, who had died in 1992.

It was not my life I was living, it was a life I was living for a dead man.

For me, losing my brain was the worst that could have happened. It was my career instrument, my differentiator, my pride, and my future. I had led my life with my brain for too long. I was finally and slowly recognizing the stress and self-neglect I had been enduring for years trying to be a wonder woman, and most importantly recognizing the fact I was not invincible. Invincibility can become imbecility. I had serious limits. At last, I recognized them. But it was OK. I finally put myself first.

Finally Turning My Life Around with Exercise and Meditation

I started running. A friend helped me. She forced me to go running almost every day. I discovered meditation with a Korean teacher, which connected body and mind as an indivisible entity. I also experienced a creative revival that I channeled into cooking at home. I came back to my roots. I cooked like my grandmother had taught me in Normandy, with fresh ingredients and many vegetables. My nutritional studies helped me understand what I needed for brain health, such as vitamins B, Omega 3, and magnesium. I lost a lot of weight and began to exit the vicious eating circle I was trapped in. I noticed sugar cravings became far and few. I experimented with the first CogniDiet® program, on myself like a Guinea pig, without knowing it. I was finally linking body and mind with caring nourishment at every level.

Eating properly, eliminating all that sugar, meditating, and running not only saved me, but gave me the courage to change; they enabled a life transformation by rewiring my brain. As I peeled off the layers of my issues, I shed the pounds. This new lifestyle triggered the endorphins and serotonin I needed, but without the sugar! They created new circuits of happiness and confidence in my brain. I am a big believer that this depression, after all, was the best thing that ever happened to me.

Meditation must be practiced, and I had ample time when I was home during my disability leave. I spent hours meditating some days. Meditation is not a trance or being in another plane all the time. You come in and out of this transcendental state frequently. I rarely speak about what I experienced because others could think I am crazy. Meditation transports you outside your body. You are one with the universe, or with God. You become just a particle, one atom, and you are, and feel the energy of everything around you. You are literally vibrating. I was able to move energy in my body, raise my body temperature, and slow my heartbeat. I couldn't achieve this every time; I learned I had to let it happen. I could not choose to make it happen. I had visions and went into past lives. I don't know if it is true, I am a rather skeptical person. Maybe deep meditation feelings and visions are just a trick from the brain. But whether what I experienced was true or not, it opened a whole new world to me and left me appeased and stronger. I let spirituality enter my soul.

With the help of meditation I started to acknowledge my limitations, but also recognize some new powers. I became gentler with myself. I became gentler with others. I also finally accepted I had to find a new life. I continued to take medications for a long time, I had small relapses, but each time, I learned to get back on track. I also completely understood the power of food. I became attuned to what reactions certain types of nutrients were triggering in my body. I understood that eating food, and especially addictive foods, is not the answer to any problem. I realized that the pleasure triggered by a doughnut was fake and temporary. I became more mindful when eating. It helped I was at home, solely focused on my health during these months. Not a luxury for everybody. But there are ways to change, even with a fully booked lifestyle. My clients are the proof of it.

I followed a complicated and sometimes contradictory road to my current life. Big changes take a long time to set in place. Maybe I am a slow learner. I know that I have always been afraid to fail. That fear was in my way for many years. But the more drastic the mutation, the longer the journey. My road was long; I had to completely change, and I was 50 years old!

By age 50, the brain wiring and habits are very profound and resistant to change, including self-image, reputation, social standing—what the world thinks of you. But you have to go above and beyond that. And your family and friends may not like it. It is very frightening to see somebody you love completely change. But a self-reinvention is also so inspiring, including to those around you.

I left big corporate America in 2009 and went into smaller, start-up pharmaceutical companies. I was training myself to be more hands-on and self-sufficient. This was a good school to prepare me for entrepreneurship.

My Own CogniDiet® Journey Is Born

In 2012, I started to write the first draft of The CogniDiet® curriculum. It had been sleeping in the back of my mind for too long. Yes, it was like a very long pregnancy! I was seeing clients in my first nutrition practice in Princeton, NJ, but realized I was not really helping them by just giving them diet protocols and calorie guidance. It is very easy to deliver an eating plan. It is another thing for the client to embrace and follow it, and by doing so in parallel, adopt a new life style. I realized that I had to help clients move from a vicious to a virtuous circle, with a focus on self-discovery and loving nourishment. You need a healthy body to undertake a mental transformation, and vice-versa. Frustrated, I studied cognitive behavioral therapy and read a lot about brain changes and neuroplasticity in order to help my clients succeed.

I have become a better person because of my new profession. More open, more attuned to others' needs. More sensitive. I let more of my feminine aspects come out. I started to record and analyze my dreams. I allowed spirituality to guide my life, not just my logical thoughts. I started to look at vegetables with a new eye. We take them for granted. They are beautiful, growing out of nothing, with the help of nature: A miracle created by God or the universe to help us thrive and grow.

Only a deep depression, a focus on mind-body balance, a back to my roots diet, and a complete reassessment of my life's vision and goals allowed me to become a new person. And only the well-nourished person I am now can be the good nurturer and guide for women and men seeking help. Transforming nutritional habits demands a serious lifestyle change. It requires courage, determination and deals with deeply ingrained habits, personal issues and pre-existing notions. I do NOT believe in diets. They fail. We don't really change.

Think about it. Nutrition literally means what "nurtures" your body and mind. It is what sets up your overall health, energy, mental balance, and ability to age well. It can counterbalance, even change, some DNA pathways. A simple vitamin deficiency can trigger diseases. Addressing the issues behind weight gain and uncontrolled eating goes deep into what we are able and willing to do for ourselves. After years leading The CogniDiet® and helping hundreds of women, I have witnessed multiple life transformations.

In 2013 I was mentally ready. I took the decision to leave my last employer and start the CogniDiet® while consulting part-time, a lucrative and less risky way to support my new business and my family. I knew as a nutritionist it would take time to build a reputation. I also wanted to learn and adapt—and manage my stress level. In fact, it took more time than I had counted on. I had found a way to live my dreams while still respecting my family obligations. I have been off anti-depressants since 2011. I haven't had a panic attack since 2008. When I feel blue, and this happens in the winter, or sometimes when I am discouraged with my business, I go back to my

B vitamins—they really work—and meditation and positive thinking. Not that I would encourage anybody who needs to take an anti-depressant not to take it. What works with me may not work with you. Anti-depressants are life savers. I truly believe that.

I am putting myself first. I am 30 pounds lighter and more muscular. I look better now than 15 years ago. No more fatty liver. I am full of energy. I know I can inspire others.

An old friend from my corporate days saw my new picture on LinkedIn® in 2016 and said, "I can see your soul shining through your eyes. You look younger, healthier and happier!" Is my life easier now? Not really, because being an entrepreneur is always risky and very time consuming. It is also kind of illogical or crazy to start a company at 55. But there is a major difference from the corporate world I left. Compassion and empathy are allowed in my new profession. This is what nurtures my soul. The extra 30 pounds, the unhealthy eating, the lack of self-care were a results of not really loving who I was.

Join Me on Your Road to Freedom from Diets

Now, a word of caution. This is my story, this is my life. Yours does not have to be as dramatic. You do not need to leave your job, move to another country, or revolutionize your entire lifestyle to become healthier and more fit! But come to think about it, something needs to change if you have been carrying an extra 40 pounds for the past 20 years and you bought this book.

I help people directly. I touch their lives. I create tears of joy and smiles and laughter. I hold hands. I listen to stories. I create supportive communities. You are not alone in your weight loss quest. You are not so different from others. You face the same challenges. That joy is the best thing I could have found in my life. I am finally me. I let my heart out. I want to help more women and men. This is why I am sharing this story. If I could transform and finally put myself first, you can, too. And you can also have fun while you are at it, unlike myself who had to do it the hard way.

Follow me on a road that will help you change your thoughts and behaviors to get in control of your eating habits and by doing so attain optimal health. And also, yes of course, lose weight and keep it off. The weight loss is the bonus. My clients often say at the end of the program they feel free. Women at one point were burning their bras in the 60's to express their need for total freedom. Well, I am not going to ask you to do that. Just dump the freaking sugar in the bin. When you are free of the burden of constant dieting you can focus your energy on achieving bigger things. If you can tame your cravings, you can tame your life. Everything is connected. Everyone is connected, too. This is why I encourage you to embark on this program with a few friends. There is a weekly group discussion guide at the end of each chapter to help you lose weight together. The road will be much smoother.

My friends, have fun, have a blast: We only live once. My personal CogniDiet® aha moment was that once I decided to get rid of the words "restrictive diet" in my life, and started to eat healthy and reasonably 80% of the time, I lost the weight.

And remember, you can have an ice cream, you can enjoy a cocktail or a rich and sumptuous meal. But the next day, get back in the saddle. This was Jackie Kennedy's rule.

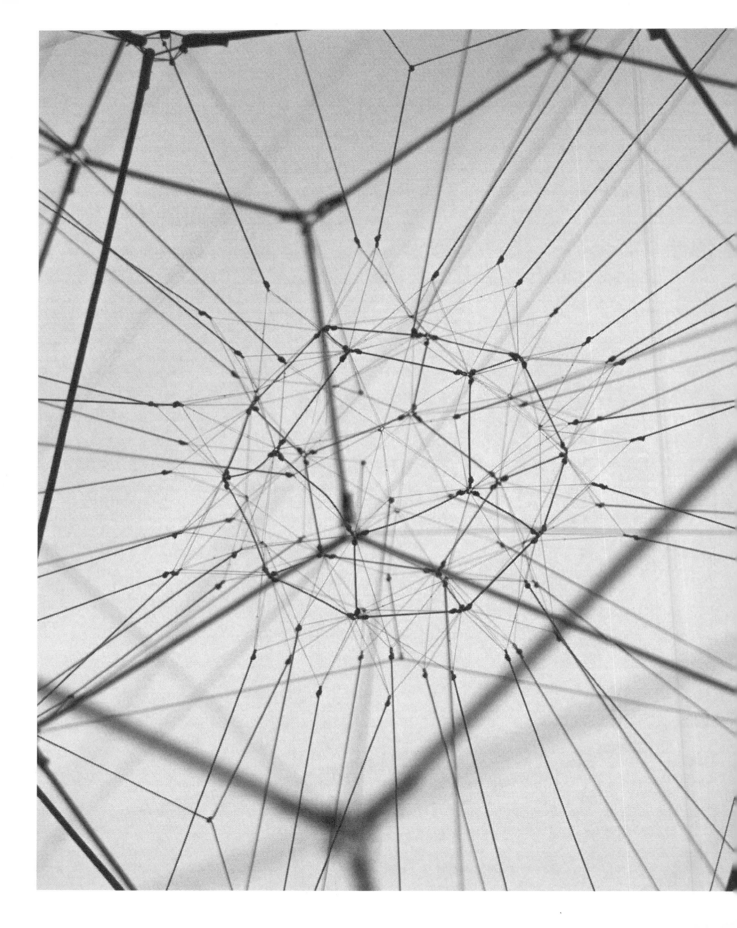

The Science
of Brain Rewiring

Your Body Will Do What Your Mind and Heart Want!

People always ask what is different about The CogniDiet®. Is this just another new diet with a smart catchy name? I have tried so many weight loss programs, why would this one be better?

You bought this book and still feel ambivalent, right? At the same time, you are hopeful you found a solution, but you are also somewhat incredulous. Can I really change my thoughts, therefore my behaviors? Can I change my lifestyle? Does weight loss really start in my brain? How can I do that?

Yes, I can help you rewire your brain, but you will have to help yourself as well. This program is for smart women who want to try something different. You are at that point where you've tried everything. You lose the weight but it comes back with a vengeance. You watch yourself going back to the pizza, the processed foods, or the sugary drinks after a few months of quasi-religious abstention. You are astute enough, deep down, to know the old tricks will not work anymore and you have to face the reality of your current lifestyle. This lifestyle so far has not supported your ideal weight goals. On the contrary, you keep on packing the pounds. I always warn potential clients that in my program there are:

✓ **No miracle pills**   ✓ **No special supplements**
✓ **No shakes or special foods**   ✓ **No points or calorie counting**

The only way to keep the pounds off is to change the way you think, eat, and move. There is no other way. It does not mean there is a life ahead of you made up of deprivation and self-denial. Absolutely not! But ahead of you, if you follow my guidance, is a more controlled life.

Let me invite you to enjoy this book, be inspired, and initiate your own nutritional and mental transformation. Take the road at your own pace, allow yourself a few detours. You can also rewind and come back to a chapter, or stay on one for longer. But there is a pedagogic and logical sense to the chapters' flow, although the first three chapters must be read first as they are the foundation of the program. After that you may decide to select chapters in a different order. You can also decide to take a break after the first six weeks and reassess your progress. Maybe you need to reboot, take a break, or you are really on a roll.

Who Is This Program For?

I also want to give you gentle advice to really benefit from this book. You have to be at that point in your life where you know, deep inside, that something needs to change. Don't wait for a nervous breakdown like me! You know this program is for you—check the boxes below if:

☐ **You have tried to lose weight forever**

☐ **You are yoyo dieting and keep on gaining more than you lost last time**

☐ **You recognize this weight is impacting your health, and your life**

☐ **You have tried every diet, bought every book, and eaten any crappy supplement, shake or processed foods that promised rapid and miraculous weight loss**

☐ **You may have tried prescription drugs**

☐ **You are tired of diets!**

You tried everything, and yet those 40 pounds are still there. No more cheating, negotiating, postponing, self-denying, or self-commiseration. No more starting and failing again and again. Girlfriend, take the bull by the horns and just do it! There may be tears, frustration, discouragement, but there will also be plenty of joy, amazing self-discoveries, surprising victories, and a wonderful blossoming of the body and the soul along the path. The CogniDiet® can support you in multiple ways beyond this book with Facebook®, Pinterest®, Instagram®, Twitter® pages, a newsletter and a webinar series. We now provide an online, accessible on demand program, in six-week increments to help women who can't come to our classes in Princeton, NJ.

There is no right or wrong. I have witnessed women losing five-15 pounds the first week (yes, it is true, I had a couple of clients who eliminated all processed foods and sugar and lost 15 pounds in one week. A big portion of that weight loss was water, however it remains impressive) and some only starting to lose weight after four weeks. We all are different and have specific body and mind resistance mechanisms in place. Some of us have stronger "knots" of old habits built in our brain. Some are truly more addicted to sugar or processed foods. Some entanglements require more patience and practice to detangle. Some of us are literally polluted by certain foods and need to clear the way first. But persistence never fails.

The CogniDiet® Philosophy

The philosophy and methodology of The CogniDiet® is to redirect the attention and focus from dieting, counting calories and banning certain foods — which equals restrictions — to YOURSELF, which means limitless self-love

---

By this I mean I want you to feel and understand how your body and mind transform with dietary and life style changes with the help of The CogniDiet® methodology.

I am not saying you can eat all you want, you will also have to make changes. But by focusing on YOU rather than the diet, you begin to recognize and understand your old habits and adopt new behaviors. In fact, you will discover a new, powerful you.

The CogniDiet® can't solve your profound emotional and psychological wounds. But you can choose, in parallel with your own self-discovery, to change your general health via optimal nourishment. You can learn to love better foods. You can stop when noticing a desire to self-sabotage with a Twix®, and get over it. I call it the "take action and move on" philosophy.

You will learn to focus on yourself and become your own detective. You are embarking on a road of self-discovery and personal awareness. It is only by doing so that you will start to understand the roots of your eating behaviors and old, ingrained patterns.

Everything you do always starts with a thought in your brain. These thoughts can be there because of logic, education, beliefs or emotions. You carry your thoughts in your head, and they impact your whole demeanor.

If you feel confident, you will look confident. If you feel sad, you will look sad. Your positive thoughts will carry you on a cloud of energy and impact your entire life. After years of testing my program, receiving client and expert input, and validating it in a clinical trial in 2016, I can really say with confidence, "My program works, and weight loss starts in your brain!"

Helping Clients Change

I had been helping clients for a couple of years as a nutritionist, but I started to feel frustrated. I realized that only focusing on a diet and calorie counting sometimes worked for the short term, but at the end, my clients went back to their old behaviors. They were focused on a temporary diet mindset, giving them unconscious permission to go back to old behaviors once "the diet" was over and the weight was lost. I was not helping them really change. With only a few exceptions the weight was back, and more, a few months later. Each time a person goes on a serious diet, her metabolism goes into survival mode and has only one goal: to replenish its stock of lost fat, and more, just in case!

It's Never a Good Time to Start a Diet!

In our ever-changing environment we are increasingly surrounded by convenience food and stores, and constant advertising, usually not for salad or celery. We rush from work to social commitments and family activities without taking a break. We go through life as if in a rat race. When is there really a good time to go on a diet? When potential clients ask me about the program I often hear "now, is not a good time."

But when are you not traveling, dealing with a stressful situation, taking a vacation, dealing with family circumstances, or just socializing? When is there a good time?

Unless you stay home and get totally in control, ignore the family, or travel with your own food, you are never in an ideal situation. Life gets in your way. This is what happened to me and this is when I decided that to lose and maintain my weight. I had to be selective, disciplined and organized. *I had to be in control 80% of the time instead of only 20%.*

- ✓ **Yes, I stopped going to certain restaurants**
- ✓ **Yes, I stopped eating certain snacks**
- ✓ **Yes, I started to carry my nuts, so that I would not have to compromise when hungry**
- ✓ **Yes, I cooked more vegetables in big batches and froze them, so I had no excuses for not eating fresh**
- ✓ **Yes, I stopped wolfing down the cookies in the meeting room or buying processed snacks in the vending machines**
- ✓ **Yes, I have pretended I was eating a crappy birthday cake at the office and threw it away in the trash can**
- ✓ **Yes, I have learned to ignore the well—or not so well—intentioned colleague who brings a freaking disgusting or too delicious cake every week and dumps Halloween candies everywhere**
- ✓ **Yes, I have learned to say NO with a smile to a second serving**
- ✓ **Yes, I am feeling great about doing it**
- ✓ **And yes, people still like me!**

How did I achieve this? By applying cognitive behavioral therapy (CBT) techniques, rewiring my brain and being cognizant of my challenges, which we will teach you in this book. My top five challenges were:

1. **Frequent business meetings with bad foods, all the time, everywhere**
2. **A sugar tooth that went into full throttle when stressed out**
3. **Too much travel**
4. **Not exercising (at least before my nervous breakdown)**
5. **Too many excuses!**

Identifying your top challenges will be essential as you embark on this adventure with me.

What are your top challenges? *And don't mention TIME!*

_____

_____

_____

_____

_____

_____

_____

_____

What Is Cognitive Behavioral Therapy?

CBT has been widely studied and proven effective in thousands of clinical trials and is used to promote behavioral changes in people with many types of issues: depression, ADHD, anxiety, anger, high stress, weight loss, disordered eating, and more. It really helps to reboot your brain.

Decades of neuroimaging research has shown that CBT produces changes in brain activity (cerebrally and subcortically) that are essentially identical to those produced by antidepressants.[1] As I underwent psychotherapy during my depression, my therapist told me I was getting anxious to the extreme because I was always imagining catastrophic scenarios for the future. The root was extreme anxiety triggered in my childhood by my parents' divorce and the uncertainty I faced every day about my future.

My therapist used a form of CBT to get rid of my pessimistic thoughts, reflect on my successes, find solutions and de-dramatize the future.

．．．

I went from:

"I am depressed, therefore weak; on a medical leave, therefore my career is compromised and I am not worth anything anymore."

to:

"I will get better with all the help I have; I am learning new tools; I am taking this break as an opportunity to take care of myself. I have had tough times in my life before, but I always managed. I am 80% happy and very fortunate. I will go back to work rested and stronger."

．．．

And I did. I just refocused my energy.

Old ideas and choices, created years ago, if not altered, will continue to drive you to the same old roads, including the same old, failed weight loss attempts. How many times are you going to count calorie points again? How many nights are you going to sip a crappy, chalky artificial shake or eat processed packaged foods?

Source 1: Baxter, L. R. (1991). PET studies of cerebral dysfunction in major depression and obsessive-compulsive disorder. The emerging prefrontal cortex consensus. Annals of Clinical Psychiatry, 3, 103—109. Baxter, L. R., et al. (1992). Caudate glucose metabolic rate changes with both drug and behavior therapy for obsessive-compulsive disorder. Archives of General Psychiatry, 49, 681-689.

I decided to apply this technique in our curriculum. In this book you will learn to transform your deeply ingrained **Sabotaging Awful Thoughts (or SATs)**, as I call them, into new **Positive Amazing Thoughts (or PATs).** Let's learn and repeat them now; you will read these two acronyms many times in this book.

I have not invented anything. Many books have been written about CBT and weight loss. I myself attended a training session with Judith Beck, Ph.D., founder of the Beck Institute for Cognitive Behavioral Therapy in Philadelphia (www.beckinstitute.org). She has written many amazing books about CBT and dieting and has been an inspiration for me. I met her as she was leading the class, and had the honor to also meet her father, Aaron Beck, M.D., who is recognized as one of the fathers of CBT. I worked on this book with Clifford Lazarus, Ph.D., a specialist in CBT and Director of the Lazarus Institute. His father is Professor Arnold Lazarus, a pioneer in multi-modal therapy and CBT as well. I also experienced my own CBT with my psychotherapist.

With The CogniDiet® Program you will learn to develop new PATs. You will write them, you will read them, you will visualize them every day. They will be tailored to your specific issues and will strengthen your power to say NO in even the most challenging situations. I will help you with experiments and games to encourage self-discovery of some of your deepest habits.

You will shift your energy from a negative pathway that will continue to set you up for failure, to one that will illuminate your brain with positive energy.

Then practice, practice, practice… I always say in my classes that I am like a piano teacher or a tennis coach. I give you the tools, the encouragement and the little tricks. But if you leave the class and do not practice, you will never progress. I myself rewired my brain after my depression with the help of CBT among other things, by focusing more on the positives aspects of my life. And it worked.

Cogni-Tip:

It is not enough to **THINK** about and formulate new PATs, you have to **TAKE ACTION!**

Once you start practicing, and there will be challenges and setbacks, you will become better at being in charge. You have to put all the positives about losing weight, and you will do this Chapter 1 in your own vision board, and balance this deep desire versus the short-term pleasure 'n get from yet another treat that you do not need.

Once you start to think differently, you start to act differently, and as you act differently you create new pathways in your brain. I became fascinated with this science only lately as I was developing my program. The idea behind this is called brain plasticity or the ability of your brain to learn new things, and change. The scientific word is neuroplasticity and as CBT, it is applied to many therapies helping people to cope with challenges such as anger, trauma, pain, etc.

Stop Thinking: "I have always failed, and women cannot lose weight after 50."

Because this thought will block your success. It's an old wiring.

Replace This Thought With a New One: "I can do it this time, it's never too late to succeed. I am doing this for myself, I deserve it."

As you put action in motion, and repeat, you are creating a new behavior and brain pathway.

And Here Comes Neuroplasticity

There is also the science of positive neuroplasticity and I have enjoyed and learned a lot about it, attending courses by Rick Hanson, Ph.D.. He has really inspired me. Check his website http://www.rickhanson.net/.

CBT is definitely linked to neuroplasticity. And yes, your brain can change even at 70 years old. The cells in your brain are mostly neurons. You have almost 100 billion neurons in your brain. Every action that you perform in your daily life involves the activation of thousands, if not millions, of neurons.

For example, think about getting out of your car. Your brain is receiving and analyzing thousands of pieces information at the same time and firing back commands. You do it automatically, right? Open door with left hand, move left leg first, then right leg, push the butt up, be careful with the door frame etc. This is the basis of neuroplasticity. Your neurons are firing, they have created a wiring. You get out of your car automatically. This is an acquired pathway. But it was created first.

Any learning must always result in changes to the brain, and for these changes to happen the brain must be plastic, which it is. The term that neuroscientists use for this malleable quality of the brain is called "plasticity". The more often we do things in sequence or together, the more the neurons responsible become accustomed to firing together.

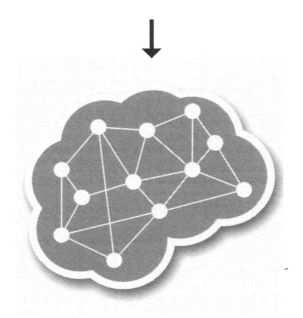

You create a new brain pathway.

INSTANT Cogni-Shift:

Now, immediately, and spontaneously, create one new pathway, let's say a new habit, that you want to implement **TODAY** (could be food, exercise or stress related)

A last element of the science that we incorporate as well in our program is the fact that the brain likes to get engaged in multiple ways. Your brain wants to have fun. Your brain likes to be stimulated. It is called "multisensory learning." It is a process that has been previously defined and explained. Are you ready to change now?

The Art of Stimulating Your Brain

Research shows that if you describe a food, the choice of words will illuminate different parts of your brain by association. An example is the use of the word "velvety." Describing a cake as simply "delicious" will not have the same impact on your brain as describing it as "delicious and velvety." The word velvety triggers memories and sensations associated with your sense of touch, and the fabric velvet. Feelings of smoothness, softness, and other words and sensations associated with velvet will also come to mind. The food and restaurant industry knows that very well. Very creatively described choices on a menu will make you salivate and anticipate the dish with impatience; words such as scrumptious, delectable, mouth-watering, golden, creamy etc. They are manipulating your brain.

Well, we will do the same! But in reverse. When you embark in some of the experiments we will share with you, it will be crucial to leverage sensations, words and descriptions that involve all your senses: touch, hearing, sight, smell, and taste. Be imaginative. I may ask you to take a turnip and look at it with tender love! Or sniff a fennel, enjoy a healthy meal and recognize the spices used in the recipe. Admire the colors in your plate when there are many vegetables vs. processed foods that are generally in the brownish, yellowish and beige palette.

The CogniDiet® Program has created fun brain games and situations experiments that will help you rewire your brain and create new circuits of happy behaviors. Alongside CBT, neuroplasticity, stress relief and nutritional education, you can really learn to change old behaviors.

Are You Ready to Change Now?

You can have wishful thinking and contemplate change. You can also take the first step. Truthfully, this is part of the evolution journey, and it can be long or short depending on multiple factors that pertain to your personality, risk tolerance factor, education background, financial situation and so much more. It took me almost 10 years to start a new career, but I took the first step by enrolling in a nutrition program.

These are the phases you will experience on your way to "change." It's called visualization, (imagining or thinking in pictures) not ideation (which typically refers to thinking in words or self-talk).

In CBT stages of change are usually referred to as:

1. Pre-contemplative (not really thinking about it)
2. Contemplative (thinking and visualizing about it)
3. Preparative (self-explanatory)
4. Active (taking actual behavioral steps, i.e., changing thinking into action)
5. Maintenance (self-explanatory)

In this program we will help you move along your road to re-invention. If you feel you are not ready, don't despair. Your time will come. I always say that just making one simple decision first, like just eliminating one food, can get you in the saddle. This small first step will encourage you to continue.

Not ready ┈┈➤ Somewhat Ready ┈┈➤ Want more Information

┈┈➤ Ready to Take a First Step

Where are you on your transformation road? Put an X on the arrow.

Whatever your "change readiness" factor is, what is a first step you could take to lose weight? I cannot emphasize enough how important the "small steps" strategy is. One small step at a time makes the change bearable, achievable and realistic.

If your new PAT is "I will not have these sugary 500 calorie coffee concoctions anymore in the morning for breakfast (and later again!), that is my first step," what will be your action? There are different approaches:

- **Go cold turkey:** Eliminate this drink totally, and replace it with a 200 calorie cappuccino with a small amount of sugar, or none
- **Downsize:** Eliminate the largest size coffee, and choose the smallest size
- **Downsize even more:** Go from coffee three times a day to once a day
- **Find a new solution:** If you realize that caffeine triggers new sugar cravings (and it does), replace it with herbal tea, or decaffeinated coffee, but do not replace it with another sugary treat!

You will reinforce your new pathway by writing in your diary: "I have eliminated approximately 10 drinks or 10 times 500 calories = 5,000 calories in my life every week. Wow, I never realized these drinks were so calorific. Good for me!" And after a few weeks, this will become a new healthy habit. You have created a new behavior. This is your first victory. And you will learn to savor your sugar free coffee. I learned to do this. I hate sugary coffee now. Even when I am stressed out! I told you earlier that stress makes us fat because stress makes us lose our head and also physiologically trigger sugar cravings. This is why stress has such importance in this book.

Looks like Stress is Derailing My Positive Amazing Thoughts!

What I have also noticed in my life and around me, is that stress is the biggest saboteur of best intentions. This is where I go one step beyond just CBT and neuroplasticity. Stress influences your logical decisions and behaviors and it is usually in a time of stress that relapses occur. An interesting fact is that my second clinical trial cohort in 2016 occurred not only during the holiday season from September to December 2016, but also during the Trump/Clinton presidential elections. My participants got out of control just before and after election week, worrying, stressing out, lamenting or celebrating. I saw weight gain and lack of control during these weeks and got worried about my trial results!

Nowadays stress is constant. And stress makes you fat. Stress used to be triggered infrequently, by the rare wild beast attack, violent thunderstorm, or the like. The brain evolved to respond to these threats with the flight or fight reaction. Then, when the threat subsided, the brain would settle back to a quieter state. But now stress is triggered nonstop. It is the never-ending commute, the holidays shopping, the security at the airport, the looming deadlines at the office, juggling family and work, you name it. However, flight and fight situations and a certain amount of stress are key for survival! And some level of stress is necessary for optimal performance. Constant stress has an impact on your mental and physical health.

In a fight or flight situation cortisol and adrenaline are released to trigger a cascade of chemical reactions. Cortisol depletes you of serotonin. These hormones also mobilize glucose in the body to supply the extra energy required by the large muscles of the legs and arms. Your heart beat goes up, your body temperature rises, and all your senses get more acute. You're in a state of intense alert. But you're not actually running or fighting. You may just be stuck in your car.

That means that the extra glucose that was released to help support the physical exertion is not used up. But your brain doesn't know that—it thinks you need to replenish your stock. Plus after a stressful event your brain usually wants soothing. Time to reach for sugary foods such as candies, cookies, and chocolate! That's why stress can make you fat.

Cogni-Tip:

Stress hijacks your brain! Logic thinking goes away. **Be aware** of your stress level.

Your brain responds to imaginary situations just like real ones. Your brain is not that smart! When you watch a scary movie, you know it is not for real, but you are still scared and jumping in your seat. Adrenaline is released, your heart beat accelerates, and your palms get sweaty. Yet you know you are safe. Fortunately, the same principles of brain functioning that can get you into trouble and pack on the pounds can be turned around to work for your benefit.

When you live through a stressful or difficult situation, your brain needs a break. It naturally seeks a hedonistic, pleasurable reward. The quick and easy solution is to grab the nearest sugary snack, or even alcohol or drugs. Truth be told, we all know your brain will want serotonin and dopamine to feel good, and we also know sugar will help with that.

What you need to do instead is choose a different type of pleasurable reward, even if it's just one that you visualize. Picture a happy scene—that last wonderful family reunion or vacation in the Grand Canyon. You think about it, you smile, you may even giggle. This is where the happy visualization technique comes in.

In developing The CogniDiet® Program, I realized that just helping people develop and implement PATs and learn about healthy nutrition and exercise was not enough. I myself led a very stressful career and lived the 4 p.m. candy hunt too many times when multiple deadlines were looming. So I searched for stress relief techniques. Of course I knew about meditation and yoga, breathing methods, meditative walks, and other relaxation techniques. They are extremely effective but sometimes they require time. I wanted something people could do every day, at any time, that would work in even a few quick minutes.

Cogni-Tip:

Breathing, distractions and visualization methods are the best techniques for short-term stress relief. They may cut your cravings short.

Breathing can be done very discreetly, even in a meeting surrounded by other people. I also searched happy brain visualization methods which are again, numerous, all carrying fancy names, but all accomplishing the same goal: calming the brain or even better, distracting it. I discovered emotional brain training (EBT) developed by Dr. Laurel Mellin, Ph.D., an Associate Clinical Professor of Community and Pediatric Medicine at the University of California, Berkeley. I have attached the links to her center and publications including her wonderful book called "Wired for Joy" that I highly recommend (www.ebtconnect.net). She inspired me greatly and you will hear more about her in Chapter 5.

In the CogniDiet® Program, you'll learn one to five-minute meditation or visualization techniques to trick your brain to be happy and deflect cravings. These simple methods will give a tremendous boost to your weight loss efforts. We will cover this in Chapters 7 and 8.

To summarize, become your own detective. Notice how you behave, what comes through your mind when meeting temptations. YOU are your own actions and choices. Be responsible. Don't hate yourself, there will be challenges, but be firm and resilient. Dare to be different. Surprise yourself. Test your limits. Let's do an instant test:

Next time you close this book, measure your stress level. What is your level now on a stress scale, from zero being absolutely not stressed, to 10 being ready to jump through a window or devour a pack of Twinkies®? If you are really seriously stressed, just pause.

Emotional Brain Training — Laurel Mellin

INSTANT Cogni-Shift:

Sit down, close your eyes, breathe calmly and conjure an image, a moment that made/makes you happy. **Count to 10 slowly.** Observe what happens.

In this book, you will start to feel changes as you go along the chapters, and it will be important to record them. But let's start with your vision for yourself. Let's begin the construction! It was recommended to me when I wrote this book to inspire readers to start a book club. I thought this was such a cool idea. So here is a map for your first meeting!

CogniDiet® Book Club Discussion Guide –
First Meeting:

We recommend you not exceed eight participants, and not everybody will always come to each meeting. For each chapter, there will be a discussion guide, so that you can share and support each other while on this journey. The book club recreates the class setting I love so much. You can share healthy recipes, cook and/or exercise, and perform a few experiments together. Today it is about understanding The CogniDiet® principles. Here are a few questions you can debate today:

- **What did you learn from Veronique's life? Do you recognize yourself?**

- **Why are you here today? How many times have you been on a diet in your life? Which ones did you try?**

- **Did they work, or not, and what did you learn about yourself?**

- **Why did you decide to do The CogniDiet® Program? What are your expectations?**

- **What are your most frequent sabotaging thoughts and behaviors?**

- **What is the impact of stress in your life in general (on a scale from 0 to 10) and the impact it has on your sugar cravings? Have you even realized there is a correlation?**

I suggest that this first meeting be used to get to know each other. The real work, including vision and goals, will be discussed the next week. You may decide to have a weight scale at the home/place where you will meet.

Acquire a binder or a notebook and get in the habit of noting your observations during the next week including challenges and victories. You will bring it with your book to your meetings in the future.

It's also very important to have a portable diary to carry with you. Note your observations and thoughts immediately. Otherwise you won't remember!

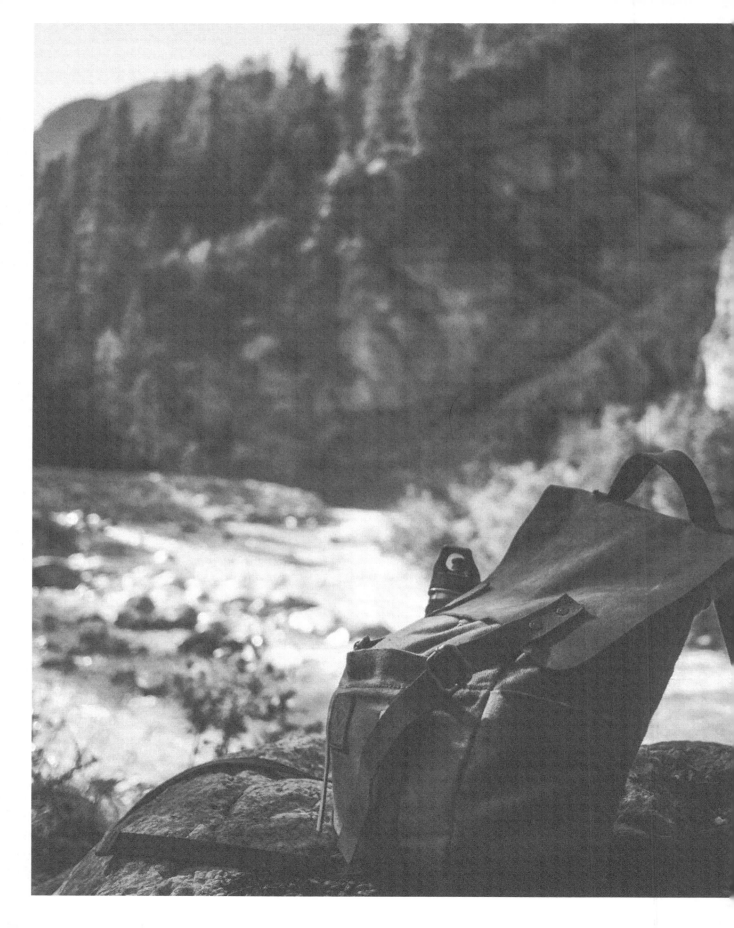

Part 1
The First 6 Weeks

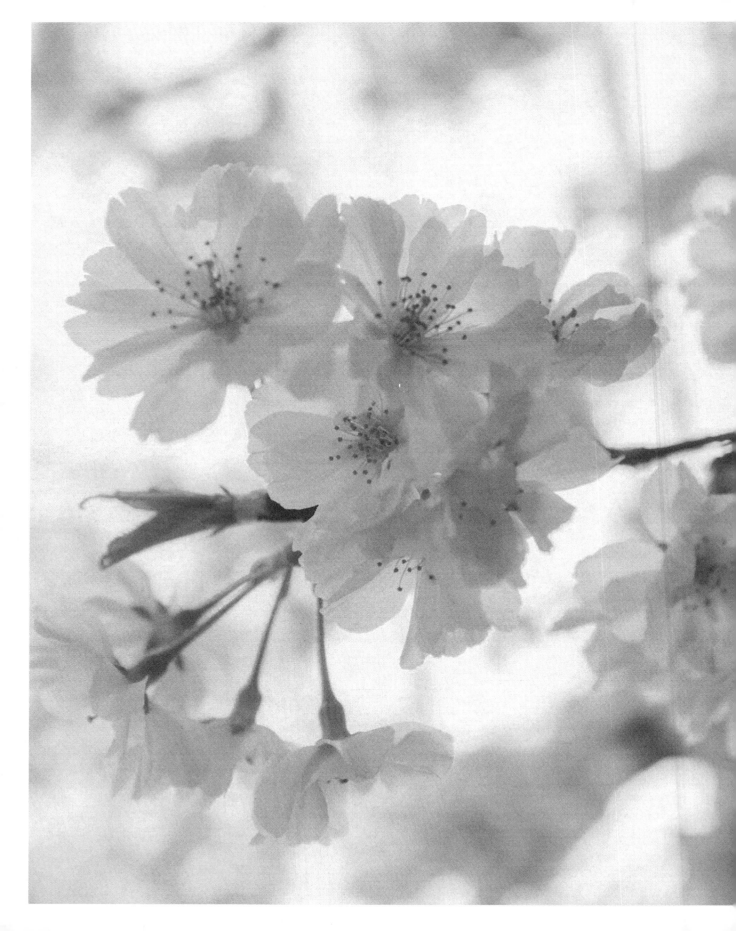

Chapter 1

My Future Me in Pictures

I Deserve to Succeed. It's My Time

My Vision Board

I will always remember my first vision board. No, it was not an elaborate creation with nice magazine pictures and colorful statements about self-empowerment. It was just in my head. It helped me stay sane as I studied for my Master of Science in Nutrition while I was at home in 2005-2006, depressed and overwhelmed. But I had promised myself I would change my life and put my soul back into it.

A new window was opening onto a new inspiring landscape, literally.

I pictured myself regularly seated at my "practitioner" desk. In my vision, I was almost always alone. Now I understand why. I was so down at that stage that I could only focus on me. The irony, yet the power of this statement, is enlightening. As I write these lines, I realize that it took a complete meltdown to allow me to finally look at and care about myself.

In this vision, I was always looking outside my office window and the view was generating a positive energy. I saw woods, trees, grass, flowers; the sun was shining a mighty light.

In my vision my space was decorated in pale wood-tones, nature based objects of decoration like drift wood, leaves, symbolic stones and plants. The whole practice was an oasis of serenity and calm.

My first real office was not like that, it was a very small, windowless room I shared with a chiropractor, but it was a first step and I felt elated. In 2013, however, my office dream was fulfilled. I had my own space with harmonious colors, pale wood bookshelves and gorgeous plants. Clients always tell me they feel at peace in my office. And it has a direct view, via three windows, to nature, and access to a beautiful garden. Yes, I see deer every evening, I have spiders and the occasional bee or wasp in the office, I enjoy the seasons and watch the trees blooming and losing their leaves. I see the snow and hear the rain. I feel the wind. Yet I am five minutes away from downtown Princeton, NJ.

I achieved my vision. It took three years to get my first windowless office and another four years until I got to the perfect one. If I could do it, you can do it too. And I lost the weight!

CogniDiet® office – View from my office
My New Life

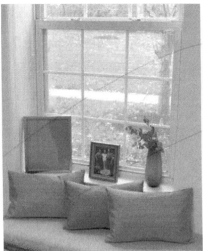

It is very important when you embark on a new quest to really figure out how you want things to play out for you. The more vivid and realistic the vision is, the more you send positive vibes to the universe that this is what you want for yourself. And the universe, I am sure, re-arranges itself to give you what you most desire. Did anyone read *The Secret* by Rhonda Byrne? Well, I did, and it helped me frame my own vision and goals.

So how are you envisioning your future life? What do you look like? Slimmer, more re-laxed, very athletic, still a brunette, still in the corporate world or surfing in sunny California? What are you doing? Where are you going? What does every day look like? These questions are very important when you embark on a new vision of you.

Have you ever really taken the time to design this new life? It does not have to be a com-plete transformation. But if your vision is to open a plant nursery along the shore in Maine, have you thought about what it would look like? The name of the company, you behind the counter or nursing a chrysanthemum patch, dealing with suppliers, wearing your large big straw hat. Yes, this straw hat that has been hanging in your garden shed for years, because you love to work in your garden and you have a gift for it.

Dream my friend, dream big, write stories, incorporate your vision in your night dreams, glue images and pictures in a scrap book, and write your own life. You will be surprised that it can actually happen. And you will also lose the weight!

Now, to be very clear, just having a vision does not cut it. If you just let it float in your brain and do not take action, the vision will stay just what it is, a nice dream. The universe will open a door for you, but you will have to cross that door and have a plan in place to venture into your new chapter. And this involves a lot of practical decisions that require planning, prioritizing and focus.

As you shed the pounds, your confidence is boosted. All of a sudden last summer, you decided to go to Maine. You followed your instincts, and your vision board. Maybe you searched plant nurseries for sale or scouted some locations. Before you knew it, you were drafting a financial plan. The vision began to turn into reality. And oh, the many signs the universe throws at you. What is it called again? Is it synchronicity? All of a sudden, you meet the perfect real estate agent by pure serendipity, at a lobster shack. He happens to be a flower expert. And your house in Ohio, where you live, that all of a sudden somebody wants to buy…speak about the universe opening its door wide open to your aspirations. Same is true for your weight.

How to Start My Vision Board

Vision board creation is a very well know technique used in many instances for life changing workshops, career re-invention, etc. It inspires a burst of energy initially. People leave the workshop completely gung ho and determined. But then the magnificent board is either hidden somewhere with no easy access, or discarded and forgotten. Or, like me, you look at your board for a very long time because you are slow to move. But as I said earlier, change is put in motion at your own pace. Your readiness factor must be ripe.

As you create your board, sometimes, interestingly, as happened with one of my friends, you forget to put in it what you desire most, and focus instead on more mundane goals. Maybe because you are afraid to face your deepest desires. This friend wanted to get love back in her life, but her vision board did not contain anything symbolically representing this with pictures such as a heart, a man, a couple, an embrace or just a big word "LOVE." It was after the fact that she realized that this crucial element had been buried under ten pictures of vegetables and fitness buffs! She said:

"I want love back in my life, I am so lonely. I am eating sweets to quiet my loneliness. But my life is not just about eating salads and carrots. My life is being vibrant, energetic and attractive. The carrot is just the means to lose weight and become healthier. I now realize I put nothing about my life's strongest desires on this board."

Pat (not her real name), 59 years old, class of 2016

In the CogniDiet®, I always start the program with a workshop to help you create your own vision board. Granted, its primary goal is weight loss. But as you know deep inside, your weight is a reflection of what is going on inside. The board helps solidify the goals you want to achieve on our 12-week program and centers on your vision as a new you, living a different life style regarding these 5 pillars:

- Food and nutrition
- Health and wellbeing
- Exercise
- Stress relief
- Purpose in life

How Do I Feel When I Change?

Think about yourself. In 12 weeks, or a little bit earlier, you are leaner. You feel your clothes hanging loose on you. Like Sharon, my first client, said one day, "I am shopping again in my closet."

Your skin is improving, your waist is getting more defined and the fat rolls are disappearing. Your legs are getting slimmer, you can feel this in your jeans. You wake up in the morning with more energy and the daily weigh-in shows steady progress. Every week you discover a new recipe or a vegetable you had never prepared before. You feel the impact of all these good nutrients in your body. Your mind is clear as crystal. Your friends tell you that you have a new bounce in your steps. And yes, it is so much easier to unload the car after shopping,

The breasts are shrinking, oh yeah, that is unavoidable, but suddenly it is easier to carry your child. You catch yourself looking at the mirror more often. You start to think about a new hair color, or maybe a new wardrobe style. Maybe going back to dating, why not? You have put a picture of an inspiring woman your age on a bike on your vision board. You plastered your board on your bathroom mirror (this is what I did with my vision board). And every day, you feel like you are starting to look like her. You even bought a yellow sweater like the one she is wearing on the picture.

Cogni-Game:

Feel the feelings of **YOU** slimmer and healthier. What are these feelings? Remember to involve all your senses as you try to find the adjectives and you envision yourself. Be bold and daring, girlfriend!

Here are a few examples of adjectives:

Beaming
Sexy
Sensual
Glowing
Attractive
Regal
Smoking hot
Alive
Confident
Joyful
Hopeful
Anew
Content
At peace
Freakinglydeliciouslyhealthy!
(I could continue this list forever.)

Feel these feelings very deeply inside your heart and mind. Close your eyes and see yourself looking the way you will look, what you will be doing at that moment, gorgeous with your yellow sweater. Maybe you are also pruning a tree in a nursery in Maine, with a cute man or woman at your side!

Cogni-Tip:

These feelings, when visualized internally and often, create a **happy brain** with **new wiring!**

Your brain is literally glowing with joy. We would see it on an MRI. When you create these positive feelings, you live them as if they are real. Your brain is being fooled. You make these feelings and emotions come true. You create new neuronal connections, you fire endorphins. You design a new neuro-roadmap. You have that power!

What are your words to describe your new feelings about yourself? Be bold!

_____

_____

_____

_____

_____

_____

What Do I Need to Start My Vision Board?

Your new feelings and look, and the life style you want to lead, will be incorporated in your vision board. So it is important to take a break and put your scissors down before you embark on your master piece. You may even to do a little bit of research and find old personal pictures, or the right magazines.

To build your board, you will need:

- A large piece of craft paper
- A pair of scissors
- A stick of glue
- Some magazines. You can recover them at many places like nail salons, hairdressers etc. People will be glad to give you the older versions
- Personal pictures if you wish _(highly recommended)_

And "voilà," you are ready to go. Find magazines that you like and represent what you are aspiring to become. Mix and match sports, nature, food, business, fashion and arts magazines. Some of you keep it very simple and have just a quote, some of you like multiple pictures and very busy boards!

Cogni-Tip:

Did you put yourself or something that is about you in the board? Even if it is a metaphorical celebrity, used as a role model, or an unknown inspiring woman, she has to be the new you. You cannot have a board with just lettuce, swimming pools and trees. **If you are absent from the board, it means you are not really focused on yourself.**

What Can I Incorporate in My Vision Board?

Let's stay open minded. You can incorporate other goals besides health, nutrition, and weight loss on your board. Women who come to my classes, are tired of diets that do not work. They tell me they know something has to change. They recognize, when gently pushed, that major facets of their lives must change as well, such as their nonexistent cooking skills, workaholic schedule or deeply ingrained fast food habits.

Maybe it is because they often are in their fifties and feel they are ready for a re-invention. Losing weight after 20 years of frustration always require a serious look at one's lifestyle choices. I have witnessed clients dumping a partner, divorcing, or starting psycho-therapy during or after the 12-week program. They quit a job or start a new career and life. They embark on a new travel adventure. They become mountaineers or kayakers at 65. I am not kidding. They learn to say no to what does not matter to them anymore. They are pruning their life as well as their body.

INSTANT Cogni-Shift:

If you can say no to the ice cream, you start to say no to other bullies! What/whom do you want to say no to? **Start doing it today.**

You become empowered, fearless, and more confident. The weight loss success, after 20 years of failure, becomes a major milestone achievement. The ability to stop worrying about it every minute, every day, liberates HUGE amounts of energy that can be devoted to bigger endeavors. More than once I see participants adding images pertaining to:

- New career or life re-invention
- Going back to school
- Travel bucket list
- Volunteering
- Dating aspirations
- Money and financial balance
- Personality changes like becoming more extroverted, or fun or free-spirited
- I bet there are some secret aspirations not always captured on the official board!

Cogni-Tip:

There is no right or wrong on a vision board, what matters is that it must inspire you. It is what YOU really want to be, feel like, look like, and live like. This is not about your kids, your partner, your mother, your family's vision of you. This is **YOUR VISION.**

Everybody will go about it differently. Some of you will create elaborate pieces of art, some will even buy special craft frames—they exist for vision boards with pin cushions, glass windows and golden frames. You can glue pictures, sentences or words, you can paint or draw, you can add personal pictures, including of yourself. It is YOUR board.

Interestingly, we revisit the boards after six weeks and after 12 weeks, in class or not, to see what has been achieved. More than once some changes occur. A vision board is a living thing. Not that it has to change all the time, because if so, the universe gets confused about what you want, but some milestones may be achieved quicker than others. And then you can get to the next on the list.

How Do I Visualize My Vision Board?

What is crucial after the creation of your board is the daily, or at least weekly, visualization and internalization of the board. You must get that discipline right. This board has to become part of your daily life. To achieve this, the board must be very visible. But you may be a secretive person. You may not want the whole world to know about this.

You created this piece of art and must strategize about where to put it. Here are some suggestions for the bold and the timid:

- Sharing your vision, put it visibly on a wall, somewhere in the house
- In your clothes' closet – very often a woman's decision in my classes
- Carry it in your purse or diary. I glued a mini-version in my diary for a while
- On your night table or bedroom, in a smaller or shorter version, framed
- You can take a picture of it and use it as a background screen on your phone or computer
- You can take a picture and frame it like a photograph on your desk
- You can create an alternative secret message board like the ones below

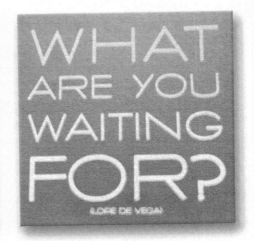

In this photo you can see inspiration boards that now hang in our CogniDiet® meeting room. Two of them have a personal story and come from home.

The first one "Go confidently in the direction of your dreams! Live the life you've imagined" was across my bed for years before I started my business. It was a reminder and an inspiration every night before sleep and every morning before a busy day that I was engaged in changing my life. And I did.

The second one "What are you waiting for" was the secret inspiration in my last corporate job. And I quit in July, 2013. It was next to my computer. My colleagues and boss thought that this statement had to do with my ability to get things done quickly. It portrayed a highly engaged, effective and committed employee. And it was true, I was working very hard and I have always been a high performer. But the true meaning was "What are you waiting for to start your own business!" This was my secret inspirational board, and I did it. By the end of 2013, my program had been piloted and my website was up. I always had a secret smile and internal chuckle when people made comments about this picture!

There is huge power in seeing your life in sentences or images. It seeps into your subconscious mind every day. I call it a positive and self-centered brainwashing. This is a message to yourself that you're control. But no vision is attainable if there is no action plan, and this is the secret to success. And for this you also need goals.

The Goal-Setting Process

I know today that I started with the vision board because I wanted to inspire you as you were reading. But this exercise goes hand in hand with the creation of your weight loss goals. I would say that the vision feeds the goals and vice versa.

Cogni-Tip:

The goals must be aligned with the vision. The goals are a means to reach the vision. The vision can be ambitious, and it should not stop you. The goals can be short, medium, or long term.

Granted that at the office we have a sophisticated medical body composition scale that allows you to target specific weight goals. But now there are some very good quality at-home scales that will give you at least your fat and water composition. For some participants, focusing on fat loss versus total weight loss is psychologically more rewarding. This scale has taught many a client that even if the scale does not budge one week, you may still have lost two pounds, but for whatever reason, you are taking medications, you ate a very salty meal, you have your periods and you packed a few extra temporary pounds of water. So you lost two pounds of fat but they were negated by an extra two pounds of water this week.

Cogni-Tip:

Splurge on a new scale that will allow you to measure body composition at home. Or use one at your gym. They often have some special body composition instruments as well, or just a manual caliper. Worst case scenario, measure your waist, hips, thighs in the middle and upper arms in the middle. Get on the scale at least every week. Set your measures as baseline and follow progress.

On the next page, you will find the template we use in our class to set up your goals. Again, I always recommend that you become laser-focused. Create your goals around our four CogniDiet® pillars:

1. Exercise
2. Weight
3. Stress
4. Nutrition

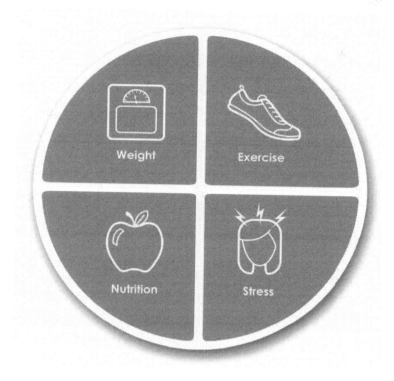

Pillar #1: Weight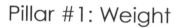

The first pillar is usually the simplest one, at least on paper! We usually recommend to have a six to 12-week goal and then, if you want, a longer term goal. I like this approach because the smaller the steps are on a long road, the more successful you will be. When clients who have been unable to lose 10 pounds over the past 15 years tell me that they want to lose 50 pounds, I always make them stop and start to ask the tough questions:

- When was the last time you lost 50 pounds?
- When you lost 10 pounds how long did you keep them off?
- Did you change anything in your life style? What foods, drinks and eating habits have you really eliminated from your diet?

INSTANT Cogni-Shift:

Leverage the theory of small steps. One pound at a time will make you achieve satisfying results week after week. It's like climbing a mountain. Do not think about the summit or the entire climb you still have to do. Look at what you have climbed already!

If you lose the weight by starving yourself or exercising to death, you are not focusing on yourself. If you lose the weight slowly but surely you are tricking your brain. There is an old man in your brain who is seated on pounds of fat. This is his treasure. He considers every pound as a golden nugget. Rob him of 50 pounds in two months and all he will want to do is replenish his coffers, and more, just in case you rob him again.

But if you steal just one golden nugget at a time, the old man may not really notice. This is our philosophy "Steady wins the race."

Cogni-Tip:

Think about reasonably losing **one to two** pounds per week. And remember, each pound lost is a victory. It becomes five pounds and then 10 pounds and before you know it you achieved your goal and lost 30 pounds. If your goal was 20 pounds and you lost 15 pounds, it is still a **VICTORY!**

Granted that if you are a big sugar addict, and you completely cut sugar the first week, you can lose as I said earlier five to 15 pounds in one week, even if it is mostly water. Yes, I have witnessed this many times. In the table on the next page, write your own goals.

My Weight Goals – Table 1

My Goals	12 Week Program	1 Year (You don't have to)	Further (You don't have to)
My weight goals: • Weight • If you have a body composition scale, have a body fat mass and % target • Or measure your body fat by using a manual caliper/measuring tape	**Examples:** I lose 12 pounds in 12 weeks or 1 lb. per week My fat loss goal is 20 pounds My % body fat is now 39%, I want to go to 31%. I lose 5in. at my waist and a total of 40in. in total.	**Example:** I lose another 20 pounds this year for a total of 36 pounds total in 12 months.	**Example:** I maintain my new weight and build more muscles

Now, Write Your Own Weight Goals:

My Goals	12 Week Program	1 Year (You don't have to)	Further (You don't have to)
Week 1			
Week 2			
Week 3			
Week 4			
Week 5			
Week 6			
Assess results			
Week 7			
Week 8			
Week 9			
Week 10			
Week 11			
Week 12			

nent, and create a weekly planner. Make sure you enter your numbers every
in your diary, or on your computer. You have to be disciplined about it.

_osing Weight

I always recommend that when you start your journey, you not only focus on the weight,
but on all the benefits you will derive from losing weight as well. Of course you have all the health
related benefits from lowering your blood pressure and lipids, to decreasing your A1c, sleeping
better by getting potentially rid of sleep apnea, etc. This is very important because it helps your
mind focus on yourself, and your own wellbeing rather than on just counting pounds lost on the
scales. Remember you have to enjoy the journey.

Cogni-Tip:

Losing weight and keeping it off means that you
create body and mind transformations that, if
enjoyed to their fullest, will trigger new "pleasure
circuits" in your brain.

Cogni-Game:

In your diary, which I highly recommend you start,
write down these benefits and come back to them
often. Describe what you really feel by losing weight.
As example of benefits I always advise you to focus
on your physical, emotional and health related
ones. Use verbs. Start with the word "I."

Here are examples of benefits, for your inspiration:

- I am able to play with my children or grandchildren again. It is amazing how much younger I look when I play with them. I feel free and joyful. I am literally beaming, running in the meadows and being goofy on the trampoline!

- I do not take a cholesterol lowering agent anymore. I have been taking it for the past 10 years. My doctor is so impressed when he saw I went from a 250 to 180 count in only a few weeks (yes this is possible!).

- I run faster now, I have noticed I am becoming lighter and it helps with my speed. I went from a 4 miles/h to a 4.5 miles/h pace in the past 4 weeks.

- I feel better in my clothes. Yes these pants are saggy now and my shoulders do not feel so constricted in my jackets anymore.

- I saw myself in the mirror, I usually do not pay attention. Boy, I felt good. I can see a real waist now!

- I feel more energetic. Usually after 4 p.m. I was getting sluggish, but now I can crank up at the office until 6 p.m. with full brain power.

- The headaches are gone!

- My face looks healthier. It is less puffy. I can see more of my features. My eyes are coming back to life. They were kind of hidden by the fat. I am using makeup again.

- I am not out of breath so quickly anymore when I run to catch my train

- I feel attractive. My partner told me I looked so good in my new dress.

- I wear a swimsuit at the beach – had not for past 10 years. I was usually wearing a beach skirt to hide my hips. But now I see definition in my thighs.

- It is amazing what a difference in my body I notice, with even five pounds lost!

- I get compliments all the time now.

Write Your Benefits:

_____

_____

_____

_____

_____

_____

_____

_____

_____

_____

Read this again and let it sink in. Close your eyes and visualize yourself galvanized by these new personal benefits. Don't you feel better already? Now you can put them into practice!

Pillar #2: Exercise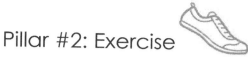

We have covered your weight goals and personal benefits, so we can now focus on your exercise goals. And yes, ladies, I will push you to move, and sweat and suffer a little bit. At the end, it is so good for us. And believe me, I am not one really jumping out of bed everyday with the adrenaline flowing because I am going to suffer for one hour with my trainer! God knows, I love him. In fact, I must give him some credit here. His real name is Luis and he has trained me since 2004. He knows everything about my life and my family. He even witnessed a gigantic panic attack and thought I was having a heart attack!

He has seen me fat, tired, discouraged. He has heard all my stories, before they became reality. I saw him fall in love, get married and have kids. I always say a trainer is like your hairdresser. The hair dresser makes you beautiful, the trainer too, but with more pain.

But he knew how to shape my body, when to push, when to be gentler, and accepted last minute cancellations after two hours on a blocked train from NYC. He was my best investment.

When choosing a trainer, select a person who knows how to work with a person your age. More than once I have witnessed 60-year-old women embarking on intense training with an unqualified trainer who thought she/he was training a 25-year-old. Make sure this is clear from the beginning. Do your homework and get feedback about this specific trainer. One unskilled trainer destroyed my left rotator cuff and brought me to a year and a half of physical therapy.

What am I asking you to do first? You may decide to tackle eating first, and keep exercise for the next weeks. In fact, it is not a bad idea. It is important to realize in the first three to four weeks how impactful nutrition is on your weight loss. This is why the chapter on exercise comes only after 6 weeks.

I want my clients to realize this first and not muddle it too much with exercising which can become a hidden compensation for an unchanged eating pattern.

But you must set some goals. You can't avoid them. When you embark on the 12-week journey, whether you are an exercise aficionado or a lazy bum, you need to be clear on what will change. I always ask initially that participants to just move it up a notch. For instance:

No exercise at all ---➤ Start walking 3 X week
Exercise 2 X week, only cardio ---➤ Add one more day of strength
Not really sweating hard on the treadmil ---➤ Increase the intensity and sweat
Bored at the gym ---➤ Discover a new sport/routine
Intimidated (yes you can be) ---➤ Hire a trainer that will educate/inspire you

What I have found works very well is when the exercise is linked to another pleasurable experience or goal such as:

- Going with a friend to support each other
- Discovering new walking trails
- Associating walking/trekking with learning about plants or foraging mushrooms
- Discovering a new cardio class with dancing involved
- Embarking on a new sport like tennis with your partner
- Going back to something you excelled at when younger, and that you remember you liked
- Biking to the office if you can
- Using a sophisticated new pedometer that allows you to compete with your friends (I do this with my daughters with my Fitbit® but always lose in number of steps as they both live in big cities)

My Exercise Goals for the Next 12 Weeks

Write down something realistic and achievable and pencil in the time in your diary!

_____

_____

_____

_____

_____

_____

Cogni-Tip:

1. Your exercising time slots must be on your calendar, week after week, otherwise there will always be a reason to occupy that time slot with something else.

———————

2. Carry spare gym attire and shoes, or a swimsuit, in your car. This is one less excuse to not stop at the gym after work.

Pillar #3: Nutrition

This section is setting your aspirational new nutritional life style for the journey. In this book I will give you information, even if condensed, that I believe you need to hear, again, or learn for the first time. But I may venture to say that if you bought this book and decided to lose weight, deep down, with all the noise that is now raised about sugar, you know that sweets will have to go. Or at least to be seriously cut. And not just because you are on a diet. No, this needs to go away because frankly speaking, it is very bad for you. It is like a monster. When it comes back, the pounds come back too—with a vengeance.

No matter how much we justify it, how many ways we try to sneak it in, you have to think that every time sugar enters your body it adds pounds, unless you are a professional athlete.

Sugar as I said, is your best friend, because every freaking part of your body loves it. The taste buds, the eyes, the smell senses, and the brain are all hooked on sugar. In fact there is a whole next chapter on sugar and this is always where I start in the program. Lose the sugar, lose the pounds. This is the only diet really. Then we go to portion sizes, and food combinations to optimize metabolism etc.

In this section I am asking you to make a few early decisions regarding:

- Your soda habits, diet or not. And yes, diet sodas still trigger further sugar cravings. Studies show a correlation between consumption of diet sodas and weight gain.
- Your fast food habits. I am talking about burgers, pizzas, burritos, hot pockets etc.
- Your sweets (desserts, snacks, drinks including sugary teas and coffees) and salty treats, usually a carbohydrate, which at the end is sugar, but with a salty flavor (tacos, chips, pretzels etc.)
- Your vegetables, and I am not talking about fries or ketchup

Take a pen and fill in a past 3-day diary of what you ate and drank. No cheating – Table 2

Day	Soda # of cans or glasses per day	Fast Food Count 1 point for each meal If you had 2 hamburgers at one meal count 2 points	Sweets/ Salty Treats Count 1 for each time you have a treat. Remember it includes sugary drinks!	Vegetables Count 1 each time you have a cup of fresh vegetables (potatoes/fries/legumes not included) Canned vegetables do not count as fresh. Frozen is OK.
Day 1				
Day 2				
Day 3				
Total				
Average (TOTAL divided by 3 days)				
Now Cut or Increase Pencil in the number	Cut by 80%	Cut by 20%	Cut by at least 80%, if not 100%	Increase by 30% or more

Then for the first two columns, agree to cut by 80% and 20% initially. I would like you to cut sweets/salty treats by 80%. For the last column on fresh vegetables...sorry guys, I want a commitment here, add 30%. This should be a good start. Apply immediately and replace the eliminated food with fresher and healthier options such as:

- A very colorful salad with a protein for lunch or dinner
- Each meal can include a protein, a vegetable, and a starchy carbohydrate such as potatoes, rice, quinoa, bread, pasta. Non starchy vegetables (could be a colorful salad) must occupy 50% of your plate, starches 25% and the protein 25%
- Snacks: fresh fruit, cut vegetables, nuts, plain yogurt instead of cake, a cookie, chips, pretzels or sweets
- Vegetables can be eaten in the form of salads, stews, soups, and green smoothies.

One word about alcohol. It is not technically sugar but it has a huge impact on your weight as well as your liver and body in general. Cut the two glasses of wine each night and you will shed pounds rapidly. Alcohol becomes sugar in your blood.

You will be surprised, even after one week to already feel your body and mind transform. You will see it again, over and over. I am asking you to eat according to the 50/25/25 plate ratio. Even when you have breakfast or a snack, or a sandwich, decompose your meal mentally and see how it would fit in a plate. Does it respect the ratio?

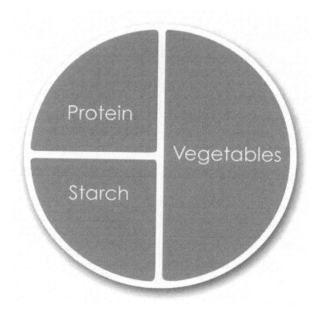

Cogni-Tip:

I always carry water with a wedge of lemon, orange, or any fruit you like. Sometimes, I even squeeze a few strawberries and pineapple in my bottle. It really gives a nice fruity flavor to my water. It replaces soda or sugary treats.

INSTANT Cogni-Shift:

Is a sugar craving coming? Count slowly to 10. Usually it will pass, or drink some water, distract yourself or walk away from the temptation. Often the body confuses thirst and hunger.

If you are already what you consider a healthy eater and not a sugar addict, then your issue must be portion sizes. Assess your portions and cut them by 20%, for each component (carbohydrates, fat, and protein).

Even if you feel you have the odd dessert or glass of wine a few times a week, it may add up at the end. A glass of wine is 120-150 calories per glass. It is technically not sugar but it kind of behaves like sugar. The odd cookie here and there adds 200 calories of mostly sugar each time also. Adopting these guidelines, which I usually call the "20% cut philosophy" will allow you to achieve weight loss very rapidly. Cutting all sugary sources can help you lose five to 15 pounds in one week. Yes, it is possible. And yes initially a great portion of it will be water.

Pillar #4: Stress

Finally, stress is also a major culprit in weight gain, one that in my opinion, we do not address enough in our society or in weight loss programs in general. The trouble with stress is that it not only destroys your health, at every level, it robs you of your perfect life, and it also makes you fat. We will cover this in more depth with practical solutions in Chapter 5.

Stress is a problem that women are more terrible at managing than men because they most of the time put everybody and everything first.

And we women feel guilty when we put ourselves first. That was my big dilemma years ago, I felt guilty if I was not with my kids, but at the gym. I felt guilty staying late at the office. But I felt guilty if I was leaving the office early, too. I felt guilty and unsatisfied most of the time. And then I realized it was because I was always caving to somebody else's priorities or desires.

You deserve and you must pay attention to your stress level. How would you describe it right now, or in general on a scale from 0 – never or little, to 10 – huge, all the time, unbearable?

What is your stress level?

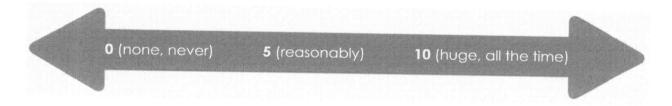

0 (none, never)   5 (reasonably)   10 (huge, all the time)

It is only when I decided to put myself first that things started to change and the universe opened new doors for me. I said I wanted to work part-time, I worked part-time. I said I wanted more time to exercise, and I exercised more often. And when I focused MORE on myself, meaning my overall wellbeing, my stress level started to go down. Why? I suspect it was due to the fact that I had taken away a lot of things I did not want to do anymore or that were creating extra stress.

What are the things you want more of in your life? Write them down. It could be more time to go back to school, more time at the gym, time to unwind or sleep more. Try to focus on new pleasurable experiences. If you want to spend more time volunteering but the responsibility creates stress, maybe it is not such a good option after all.

I have a client who decided that no matter what, she would work from home on Fridays and that would be non-negotiable. She literally imposed it to her employer, and things got organized around her not being at the office that day.

Big Cogni-Tip:

Learn to stand up for yourself:

"I started to pencil in, twice a week, training sessions at the gym. I told my husband I needed this for my own sanity and that it was not negotiable. He would have to take care of the kids these two evenings. He did. I did not ask him, I told him. He tried to sabotage me once or twice but it did not work. I told him to find a solution outside of me being the last minute savior!"

Kathleen, 44, Class of 2016

"I am a stress eliminator." This is what Lisa said in 2017, when she decided she would resign from her school PTA board. She realized it was adding unnecessary stress to her life. It was a hard decision but up to this day, as I write this book, she has no regrets. And she has lost 30 pounds.

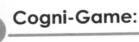

Cogni-Game:

Become a big Stress Eliminator! Take care of your needs.

What can you eliminate? Here a few examples. Look at your life every day, and hear yourself complaining that you have too much to do. Now, assess what you can let go of!

- Too many volunteering tasks

- Do you need to go grocery shopping every day?

- How much time do you spend on Facebook, Twitter or other social media (just check). It creates stress, and anxiety, believe it or not.

- Why go to three social events a week? And then have no time to exercise? Maybe one event is enough?

- Commuting back and forth four hours a day? Maye it is time to consider a job change or a move?

- Traveling four days a week – I quit a traveling job years ago for that reason.

- Horrible boss or partner? Not easy, I know. But maybe it is really destroying your life and soul. How long can you take it?

- Four restaurants a week, really!

- An hour and a half a day for personal grooming, maybe you could simplify? Think highlights, pedicure, manicure, tanning bed, elaborate make up, hair straightening…

- Not able to say no at the office and always taking over others chores, while they leave at 5 p.m.?

- Avoiding toxic situations if you can, family, friends or office related.

Let's ask yourself, if your stress level is a regular 5 to 7, what will you do to take things into your own powerful hands? What would it take to get to a 3 to 5 at least a few days a week? Or a zero at least once a week?

Can you simplify your life? Or is it that you can only change a little right now. If this is the case, what will you do to deal with your stress? Because it is not going away. It is like a cancer in your body. It inflames every cell, releases huge amounts of cortisol, depletes your adrenals, and makes your immune system weaker. And I could go on and on and on about it.

Cogni-Game:

Now Replace What You Eliminated With What **YOU** Like and Need!

Write down a few things you will do for yourself, besides what you can eliminate:

- A calming meditation or gentle yoga daily practice
- Getting the stress out via sweating in a sauna or performing gentle exercise, like swimming
- Walking in nature is proven to reduce cortisol levels and make your brain happy
- Creating little daily pampering ceremonials like a nice tea, a soothing bath, a face mask, etc.
- Aromatherapy techniques. Smelling some oils can calm you down. Try citrusy flavors
- Taking mini mental breaks. Not everybody has the luxury to have a massage. But everybody can take five minutes to relax, anywhere.

My stress reduction resolutions

_____

_____

_____

_____

_____

_____

INSTANT Cogni-Shift:

Next time you have a stressful moment, take a deep breath several times and think about your stress resolutions. What will you do today to lower your stress?

Here we are, we are finished with our vision and goal-setting chapter for this journey. Now you are clear, at least I hope, on what you are trying to achieve. It is only by taking care of yourself holistically that you can change and influence your weight. I always say your weight is a carapace. The more you are in pain, or hiding your true self, the more fat there is to protect your true core. Let's peel all the layers together, and enjoy the transformation. I am sure you discovered already a few interesting things about yourself in this chapter.

As a final inspiration I want to share the story of one of my first clients, Susan—not her real name. She was a high-level executive in a large corporation. Intelligent, articulate, a wonderful speaker and a great leader. A beautiful woman, with a heart of gold. I felt we were kindred spirits and we became friends.

Susan's Journey: The Learning of Self-Love

When Susan spoke in the class, people listened. She is extremely eloquent and articulate. I always admired her ability to unearth the deepest insights from within her soul. She had a brutal honesty about herself and courage in facing her challenges. Like me, her husband was at home most of her career, allowing her to reach her true professional potential.

But inside, her soul was almost dead when I met her. She had tried every diet. Succeeding at it for a few weeks and then going back to her old habits. She had completely left her true self behind. The mind builds a fortress around the body as a protection. And the bigger the fortress, the tougher to go back to the core of the soul and the real person that hides inside. To get out of your own self-built fortress is an act of strength and immense courage. I will never say it enough, I truly admire and respect all my clients and friends who decided one day to find a way out. For Susan, the first step was to quit her job so that she could focus on herself. This was risky but necessary. It also allowed her to explore what she wanted to do as a next career.

Cooking was not a forte in the family which relied on fast food, take-out, and processed solutions. But after attending our class, slowly but surely, the dynamics, menus, and eating rituals started to change at the family level, including with the children. There were some upsets but she kept going. She lost almost 15 pounds her first week by just eliminating sugar, processed foods and alcohol.

What they did as a family is part of the story. They got rid of all the crap. They shopped for healthy foods and attended some cooking classes. They studied labels. They cleaned the house and wiped out all the unhealthy, mostly processed foods. They got rid of alcohol, too; no more wino at dinner! The results were extremely rapid.

What she did for herself was to learn self-love. Allowing herself to receive what she deserved. She became a receiver rather than a giver.

She learned to stop before acting — on any topic — and developed a method called "What about ME?" If her ME part was not satisfied, even as a portion, she would not do it. This was her new pathway.

Susan succeeded with the help of her family. Find a friend or family member to help you, or accompany you in this journey. Do the program together. Compare your vision boards, set goals you can achieve together. You will see, it will be much easier. You will need this friend in the next chapter, because I will ask you to let go of sugar! And this is when the book club becomes handy!

CogniDiet® Book Club Discussion Guide

This week there are plenty of activities you can share with your book club. And you can set your vision and goals together. At the beginning of each meeting it is always very important to start by sharing the challenges and successes of the past week:

- Create your vision boards together, this is so much fun. Or bring yours to the discussion. The group must agree upon the agenda and some of you will be responsible for bringing the right materials and magazines if you want to build your vision boards together.

- Share a common template (Table 1 and Table 2) and discuss your goals (weight, exercise, nutrition, and stress reduction) and benefits. Find activities you could share such as:
    - Cooking and/or shopping for food together
    - Exercising/de-stressing together
    - Learning something new together.

- You may even introduce a friendly competition with prizes. I do this in my classes. These are small gifts like a nice soap, or bath salts to relax, a pedometer, a special spice, you name it...

- When you eat together, play the plate game. Eat according to the 50/25/25 ratio. Eat the vegetables first. Gauge your appetite before and after the meal

- What are your stress reduction goals? Be serious about them. What can you take off of your plate, no pun intended?

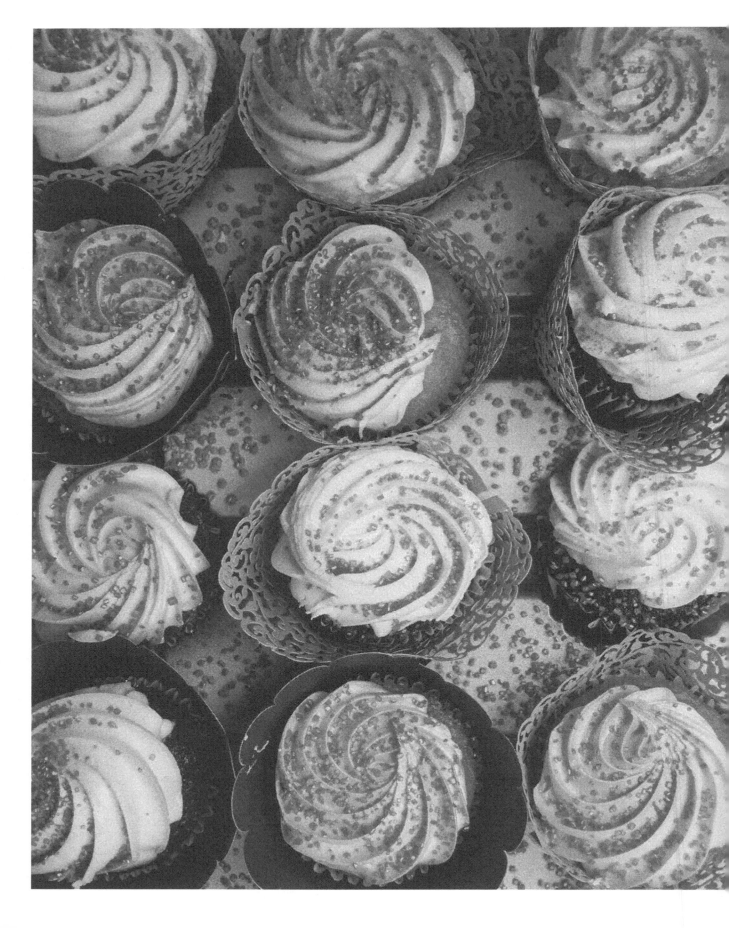

Chapter 2

I Am Getting Rid of Sugar!

Sugar Is Your Enemy – Just Learn to Dominate It

It is Halloween in our subdivision. My young girls love it and we have prepared for the event with the usual candy and chocolate single serving, multi-pack, shopping spree. They have been bought weeks in advance, because advertising starts earlier each year for such celebrations. You are encouraged to buy your candies by September nowadays. Good excuse for all of us, because the big bags in the closet have been opened, and candy is disappearing mysteriously before the big splurge day. Especially my favorites, the Reese's® peanut butter cups.

What is going on in that closet? The large size and depth of the bag is very welcome. It hides the multiple thefts. I take a few when I go to work. I take a few when I come home. Yet, I forbid my kids to steal anything. But they are smart and excited, and tempted, too. They are checking the not so secret stash. They complain it has been opened and candy is disappearing.

I am secretly eating the candies. The single mini serving is a diabolical invention because it gives you permission to pretend you only eat small portions. You can eat them everywhere. And you can hide the addiction because you are stashing it so easily, hidden in your pocket or hand. And one mouthful is so easily swallowed. Even that can be done secretly in front of a full room. I remember eating one on my way to the TV room, on my way up the stairs, and even in the bathroom! I call them the "in-betweeners," or the mini sugar breaks. Much easier managed than a piece of cake or even a cookie that requires too many bites and is too visible. It is so easy to be sneaky with mini snacks nowadays.

On Halloween night things get even more out of control. Each time the bell rings I open the door and dip for myself into the bowl. I am feeling sick. I have chocolate nausea and my mouth is sore—from all the sugar and the preservatives combined. I realize I must have eaten 20 mini bites in one day. This is almost 600 to 1,000 calories of pure processed sugar, and bad fats, or more than half my nutritional need in calories. Veronique, please; what are you doing?

This is sick. When I think about the past, I wonder how I could inflict this upon myself. What was the real pleasure? Once you start you can't stop, you are like the hamster on the wheel. One candy after the other, like a curse. Not a surprise the pants were cracking at the seams. And the belly got like jellyfish. I remember being ashamed of myself, yet powerless at breaking the curse. I am so glad I got out of this cycle. And if you follow my guidance, you can too.

If you are a sugar addict you know all the tricks, the hiding places, the deception, the games, the excuses, the before and after, the highs and the lows. You have stashed candy in your bras, in your shoes, in your car, in the garage. I bet you have been very resourceful. One of my daughters had hidden a private stash at home, after Halloween, not very smartly between her mattress and her bed board. We had an incredible chocolate Labrador called Zapper who was obsessed with food. We found Barbie® shoes, wrappers, and kids' latex balloons in her poop frequently.

Well, she found the bag and ate all the chocolates, with the wrappers. She was not even sick and we found the wrappers in her poop too!

Sugar is a cheap and available drug, with multiple flavors, sizes and shapes. I am a marketer by training. Food companies have flavor and texture engineers, consumer tasting focus panels, market research and all the necessary tools to target and hit the right consumer with the right product.

Do you prefer chewy, crunchy, salty, gooey, cold, creamy, chocolaty or peanut buttery? Maybe a combination…why not add some fizziness! That's how they hook you. They engage all your senses, including with advertising.

Cogni-Game:

> Take a piece of candy or chocolate and analyze the label. How many natural ingredients are there? Now, what are they saying in their ads?

And then you can add the three Starbucks® or Dunkin' Donuts® that are located near your home, your office, on your way to school or near your local shopping center. They are waiting for you with open arms. They can feed your caffeine and whipped cream addiction on top of everything. They are part of your daily ritual. They are a habit too, these liquid little treats.

Is this chapter going to be a lecture on sugar? I will try not to make it one. But I will share a few facts that are part of what I consider a mountain of damning evidence that should help you start to look at sugar with a very different eye. I will also offer you some solutions that you will mostly learn via our little experiments. I also recommend the very recently published book from Professor Robert H. Lustig, M.D., called "The Hacking of the American Mind" (visit his website: Robert. H. Lustig UCSF).

The CogniDiet® first session curriculum is all about sugar. Eliminate the sugar and you will lose weight fast. Sugar or carbohydrates are a source of energy. It is the fuel of your body. But it needs to be "burned" with activity. So guess what happens when you eat three cookies and then stay on a couch for three hours?

There are five facts I would like you to know about sugar:

1. All carbohydrates end up as glucose in your blood.

Some carbohydrates trigger very brutal spikes, usually the "white stuff," or pure sugar. Some, because there is fiber and some fat (think real whole grain bread where you can still see the oily kernels, or oatmeal) have a slower uptake. Remember that even vegetables and fruits, including non-starchy vegetables, are carbohydrates, but as you will see later, with much less sugar content.

Each time there is too much glucose in your blood, insulin is pumped from your pancreas to deal with the extra glucose and extract it from your blood. If there is too much glucose in the blood it leads to diabetes, heart disease and more. As a strange result of having too much glucose in your blood, your body goes overprotective and takes it out. Your glucose level drops dramatically and triggers a new craving for refueling. This is the vicious circle of sugar.

Sugar Release Patterns
This is how you create never ending sugar cravings.

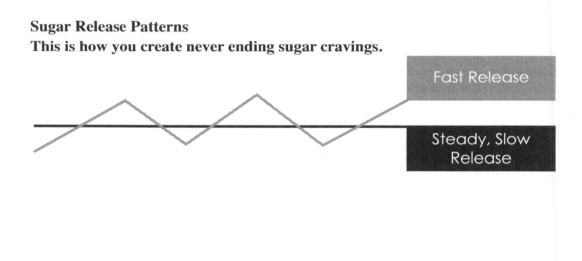

All fruits, vegetables, flours and starches have a glycemic index that measures the rapidity at which sugar is released as glucose in your blood. You will notice most of the non-starchy vegetables have low indexes or none! White stuff foods can release sugar as soon as 10 minutes.

Glycemic Index of Carbohydrates

Food Type – All 15g Carbohydrates	Glycemic Index (GI)
Non-starchy vegetables: Artichoke (1/4 cup), asparagus (1 cup), avocado (1/3 cup), bean sprouts (3/4 cup), bok choy (1 cup), broccoli (1 cup), Brussels sprouts (3/4 cup), cabbage (1 cup), cauliflower (1 cup), celery (4 stalks), cucumber (1 medium), eggplant (1 cup), fennel (3/4 cup), green beans (1/2 cup), mushrooms (2 cups), peppers (1/2 to ¾ cups), all salads (2 to 3 cups), snow peas (1 cup), spinach (4 cups), tomato (1 medium of 1 cup), turnip (1 cup), zucchini (1 cup)	GI is 0 (zero) when raw, sometimes cooking can increase the glycemic index slightly. Except for carrots (1/3 cup), with a GI of 35
Starchy vegetables: Beans in general, lentils, chickpeas, hummus, beets, butternut squash, corn, parsnips cooked, peas cooked, all potatoes, pumpkin	Between 30 and 75 (highest is white potatoes)
Fruits: **Lowest:** apple (small), grapefruit (small), orange (medium), peach (large), pear (1/2 of a large), plums (2), raspberries (1 cup), strawberries (1 ¼ cup) **Highest:** banana, apricots, cantaloupe, black cherries, grapes, mango, papaya, pineapple, raisins, watermelon	Lowest are raspberries at zero, but usually in the high 30s and 40s Highest is 75 (watermelon) to lowest mango (51)
White or whole carbohydrates: Bread (1 slice), rice and pasta, (usually a 1/3 to 1/2 cup cooked)	Between 40 and 70, more likely around 60.

Table based (and simplified) on page 344-351 of "The Best Life Guide to Managing Diabetes and Pre-Diabetes" by Bob Greene, John J. Merendino Jr., M.D., and Janis Jibrin, M.S., R.D. Simon & Shuster.

2. Ideally, the body can only process 30g of carbohydrates every 2 hours.[1]

This is what your pancreas is able to handle with insulin. Yes, even the good carbohydrates (except most of the vegetables, which are very low in sugar). Learn to picture what 15g of carbohydrates represent. It is essential to become a master at that, because this will be the number one reason you will be able to lose weight besides portion control.

The numbers below are approximate numbers. Some foods can be 16g or 13g, but I decided to simplify things for the sake of your learning journey. All sources are from MyFitnessPal®, the app that I use regularly to check my calories:

1 Serving = 15g Carbohydrates (Rounded)

- 1 slice bread, 1/4 bagel, 3/4 cup cooked oatmeal
- 1/3 to 1/2 cup rice, 1/3 cup pasta, 1/2 cup corn
- 1/2 cup cooked potatoes, 3/4 cup of fries (half a small portion)
- 1-2 cups cooked or 2-3 cups uncooked vegetables
- 1 small apple, 1/2 medium banana, 1 to 3/4 cup any berries
- 5.2 oz wine glass: 2g sugar + 15g alcohol
- 1/2 cup vanilla ice cream or a small cookie

3. If not burnt within 2 hours[2] (15 to 30 minutes for rapid releasing sugars such as pure sugary/white carbohydrate treats or alcohol) insulin transports the extra glucose out of your blood to be stored as fat.

Extra glucose beyond acceptable safe levels cannot stay in your blood. It destroys your organs. However, having 40g of carbohydrates or more at a meal is not too bad if you burn the fuel after the meal. Even your body at rest burns sugar for all the activities going on like digestion or your heart beating. And then normal activities such as walking, getting up the stairs, vacuuming or just being moderately active will burn this sugar. You don't have to jump on your elliptical. I

1 and 2: "The Insulin Resistance Diet" by Cheryle R. Hart, M.D. and Mary Kay Grossman, R.D.

am trying to say that being a couch potato or being glued to your computer after having a cake are not ideal situations! Because this is what glucose's role is in your body. You need to be active, go walking, or exercise to burn it off. This is why we strongly recommend TO NOT EAT STARCHY CARBS and SUGAR for dinner. You will always burn carbohydrates even at rest but at a slow pace and especially when you sleep!

Cogni-Tip:

Eliminate sugar and starchy carbs for a few days at dinner and you will be very pleased with your weight loss!

Insulin is a fat storing machine. Both sugar and carbohydrates make you fat—very rapidly. And fruits are carbohydrates! The only exception is non-starchy vegetables; they behave differently and do not trigger high glucose spikes (see in previous Glycemic index table).

TOO MUCH SUGAR + NOT MOVING = FAT CREATION
1 cookie = 15g or 60 calories of carbohydrates to burn

It is not just fat that makes you fat, it is too much glucose!

4. All sugars are sugars, honey!

There is no GOOD sugar. No, honey is not OK if you consume too much of it. Some sugars are just worse than others at creating even higher glucose peaks. One example is industrial corn syrup which bears many new names to fool you, and is added to almost every processed food nowadays including hams, meats, condiments, bread. The list is endless and the industry keeps on coming up with new names to hide it. A new one is "inverted sugar." In fact, yet again, it is corn based sugar.

Cogni-Game:

Become a label detective. Find the hidden sugars!

Are artificial sweeteners OK? The research has now officially linked them to many health issues and the ability to still trigger sugar cravings and trigger insulin spikes.

The next question will be: "Is stevia OK?" Stevia is a plant. It grows in New Jersey. It is bitter. The powder however has been engineered to be pure, without aftertaste. It may be combined with other sweeteners. It has undergone a chemical process. Therefore, I am not interested.

Although some nutritional experts may disagree with me, I believe everything should be eaten as close as possible to their natural form. I will not condemn sugar totally. But I will suggest that if you can't live without it, try good raw and organic honey or raw sugar in extreme moderation, added to your cup of coffee, instead of any other sweeteners. Do not exceed 4-6 extra teaspoons a day. Do we know what stevia will do in the long run to your body? Not yet.

Cogni-Tip:

My recommendation: Learn to live without added sugar. If you want some, choose a natural and trusted source.

Sugar Is Sugar, Read Your Labels!

- Beet sugar   • Cane sugar   • Agave syrup   • Honey—yes, honey is sugar!
- Fruit juices (even if it comes from a natural source, it is added sugar) and fruit extracts
- Molasses (viscous by-product from the refining of sugar cane or beets)
- Maple syrup and more
- All the "ol" sugars like mannitol and erythritol are sugars even if the food industry can claim there is zero sugar when they are added. They have a lesser glycemic index but promote gas

The worst:

- Corn syrup or fructose or high fructose corn syrup (re-engineered sugar extracted from corn starch)
- High maltose corn syrup (a new way to trick us, but it is also made of re-engineered corn-based starch)
- Dextrose (another name for sugar)
- Inverted sugar (a new way to fool you) = glucose + fructose

5. Last but not least, sugar and white processed carbohydrates (including in drinks) create inflammation in your body. They trigger all sorts of diseases beyond weight gain, such as Type 2 diabetes, cardiovascular diseases, elevated cholesterol, and even fatty livers.

We have all heard and read about the multiple nefarious effects of sugar. It is even linked to cognitive degeneration and some call Alzheimer's disease Type 3 diabetes. I want to speak about something that is getting more attention now. Something new.

Fatty liver is like French "foie gras," only you are the goose. The geese are fed high corn meal diets. Corn starches deliver glucose/fructose based sugars. These engineered sugars (even real sugar when too much is eaten) are too much to handle for the liver. The liver starts to create extra fat. Ensues a form of liver engorgement that leads to cirrhosis, only not triggered by alcohol. The end is liver transplant. Remember alcohol is also sugar, by the way.

This disease is now seen in children as well, and affects, silently, 70-90 million Americans.[3] This is because we eat too many processed foods and drinks containing mostly corn syrup, and too much sugar in general. The corn based sugar is the deadliest because it contains fructose, the most dangerous for the liver. The outcome of this is not only a fatty liver, but also cardiovascular disease, and it goes hand in hand with obesity and diabetes.

Now, you are totally depressed and guilty and feeling powerless because I just hit you with all these facts. But you need to know, you need to become aware of how much sugar you eat. You need to know what sugar does to you. If you do not like what you see here my friends, close the book and ask for a refund.

I am not telling you to stop eating sugar, or avoid all ice cream or little pleasures, I am begging you TO CONTROL and LIMIT. And try to choose good sources, as unprocessed as possible.

I am asking you to control your intake, not just for your weight loss, which cannot, and will not occur without cutting sugar. I am asking you to cut sugar for your health. You all know sugar is the Number 1 reason we have an obesity and diabetes epidemic in the U.S.

3: "Modeling the epidemic of non alcoholic fatty liver disease demonstrates an exponential increase in burden of disease" by Chris Estes et al, Hepatology, doi:10.1002/hep.29466

Weight will, for sure, 100% guaranteed, come back with a vengeance when sugar creeps back in. And by the way, a salted pretzel addiction is a sugar addiction. White flour in all its glory is a white carbohydrate and is like cocaine, as shown in studies with rats. This white powder gets you addicted.

There is no miracle pill, no special trick, and no secret sauce. You must eliminate sugar to lose and keep weight gain at bay.

THE ESSENTIAL FIVE COGNI-RULES

Apply them and win your battle with sugar:

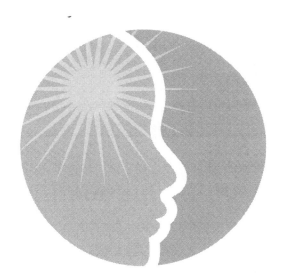

Rule #1. Always add a fat when eating a carbohydrate.

It will slow down the release of glucose and limit blood spikes, which trigger new cravings. Good fat, which we will cover in another chapter, is making a comeback. Eating good fat can help you lose weight. Yes that is an interesting truth, and will make you feel more satisfied, longer.

Examples:

- A fruit with a few (8) almonds or nut butter
- A whole grain cracker with some cheese (not an ideal snack but at least you combined)
- Oatmeal (slow carbohydrate) with some 2% fat yogurt
- A protein shake with some 2% dairy or almond milk, veggies and fruits

Rule #2: Always add a protein when eating a carbohydrate.

Linking protein with carbohydrates and fat allows for lower insulin needs, therefore less fat storing. Protein will also help you feel satisfied longer and maintain your muscle mass. Again this is a very important principle I learned from "The Insulin Resistance Diet" by Cheryle R. Hart, M.D. and Mary Kay Grossman, R.D. The snacks here above also contain protein. It is usually recommended to follow the one to two ratio or 1g of protein for every 2g of carbohydrates.

Rule #3: Favor vegetables and slow release whole carbohydrates to white carbohydrates.

Vegetable snacks will eliminate cravings because of their water and fiber content. You will feel full, yet you will not create glucose spikes that in turn will trigger new cravings. This is why you see these new recipes now using cauliflower crusts for pizzas, spiralized zucchini instead of pasta, mushrooms used as thickeners, almond flour based pastries and more. You know by now vegetables have a zero to very low glycemic index.

Rule #4: Try to limit carbohydrates to 100 to 150g NET a day to lose and maintain weight-loss.

This is approximately 400 to 600 calories in your daily intake. If you want to accelerate weight loss go between slightly under 100mg and favor vegetables, which only pack a few calories a cup as seen on previous table. And remember avoid starchy carbs and sugar at dinner. The so called low carbohydrate-high fat (LCHF) or ketogenic diet advocates as low as 20g of carbohydrates a day and an amazing amount of fat. The premise is that the body will burn fat as fuel if deprived of glucose. I do not recommend this diet unless you are very severely addicted and health impaired by starchy carbohydrates and sugar.

It is important to subtract fiber, which passes through yours system unchanged, with no calories, out of your carbohydrates count. You will see this on labels. The net impact of carbohydrates is for instance:

Total carbohydrates = 36g	
Fiber =	10g
Net carbs =	(36-10) = 26g.

Fiber is very important for your health. Most fiber-rich foods are vegetables, fruits, legumes and whole grains. Real whole grains. It can be insoluble, like these strings of fiber you see in celery stalks or avocados. The soluble fiber on the other hand forms a gelatinous mass. Chia seeds or flax seeds when soaked form a gelatinous mass. You can observe the same with oats when cooked. That is soluble fiber. **We need 25-30g of fiber (soluble or insoluble) a day** and the benefits of fiber besides lowering cholesterol and making you feel full, is that it acts as the carwash of your digestive tract. They are the cleaners and help you get rid of toxins.

....

Rule #5: Play with distractions or use a few tricks.

When the craving occurs and you want to keep it at bay, you can learn some calming techniques later in Chapter 5 covering stress. However there are other quick short term solutions like engaging in another activity such as giving a call, going for a walk, or really putting your mind into something else. There are also some nutritional strategies:

- Drink a glass of water. Thirst can be perceived as hunger.

- Chew a mint flavored gum or even better, drink a mint tea.

- Get a bitters spray (a company called Urban Moonshine sells them online). It will trick your brain with a bitter taste that may make your brain forget about sugar or squeeze a few drops of lemon on your tongue.

- Take a Chromium piccolinate tablet (go to Chapter 10).

- Have a fat bomb! By that I mean something that is high in fat, will satisfy you and will curb your cravings. For instance a few scoops of avocado or a full fat sugar free yogurt, or a few nuts.

- Have a whiff of some essential oils like peppermint oil, or citrusy smells.

This concludes this chapter, one of the toughest ones, because it addresses the root cause of why your waist is expanding every year. Eating fresh vegetables, and a lot of them, and limited whole grains, is the key to maintaining a steady level of glucose in your blood to avoid cravings, and changing your body and your health. Think about your ancestors running in the forest, hunting and eating berries and roots. There were no coffee shops, ice cream parlors or restaurants.

I now want to share the story of my dear and beautiful Sharon. She is the first person who called me in 2013 after she heard me speak somewhere about my program. Sharon is a beautiful 65-year-old redhead who had been a teacher her entire career. A devastating budget cut in New Jersey forced her to retire in 2013. She was angry, and believe me, you do not mess with Sharon. She had been a sugar addict all her life and was even a member of Overeaters Anonymous for many years. She lost almost 20 pounds when she attended our pilot program. She came back after one year to do it again, and combined with intensive training with a personal coach, she lost another 20 pounds. We are now in 2017 and she still has not regained these 40 pounds.

How did she do it? The first thing to realize here is that you can lose 40 pounds at age 62. It is never too late. You can also start to exercise and build muscles. You also can get rid of a lifetime of habits at 62! You just have to put yourself first and make your transformation a life goal. Sharon did it with bravery, steel resolve and grace.

Sharon's Story: How to Get Rid of a Sweet Tooth!

Sharon became completely in control of her own destiny, even while living with the biggest saboteur possible, her sugar addict husband. I remember she told me that her husband was eating candy in their bed while she was trying to eliminate sugar. He still offered her cookies while she was openly on the program, and she kept on saying NO. She designed a special kitchen-drawer for his foods and forbade him to exhibit them on the kitchen counter.

She traveled to Disney by car with her family for their yearly trip and for the first time in 20 years, she brought coolers with her with as much of her own food as she could for the one week trip. She mapped her restaurant choices, she asked for special foods, she told her husband and two daughters to let her live her life. She came back five pounds lighter and confessed that every year she went to Disney she usually came back with an extra 10 pounds.

On Christmas, she had to visit family members who were sugar confectioners. Their home was a fairytale landscape of sugary treats. But she felt she had entered hell. She resisted. She told me than more than once she disappeared in the restroom where she used mindful meditation techniques to visualize herself healthy and fit.

Her secret method to resist sugar was to:

- Learn what sugar was doing to her body.
- "X-ray" all sugary foods, crossing them off her list mentally with a big red X. Or visualize the word POISON or TOXIC written on it.
- Change her eating habits. Adding more slow carbohydrates and vegetables, link foods and never compromise. Even at weddings or parties, she chose the healthier options or called in advance to make sure there were special meals. She told me "every day counts."
- Eliminate certain restaurants and swipe her house out of temptations. Even her husband had to hide his stash.

In the process of doing these steps, Sharon also found a new career as an Adjunct Professor at Penn State University. She is training future teachers with passion and expertise. She chuckled as she told me how over the past years, while she maintained her weight loss, her girlfriends yo-yoed up and down. They always ask her for her secret, hoping there is a magic pill. She answers that she just decided once and for all to be in charge. She shared her PAT:

"I am the boss of myself, the only one. Nobody can tell me what to eat!"

Now, let's introduce our first Experiments Series, for the body and mind, that will allow you, over the course of this book, to self-discover and transform your life every week!

Experiment #1 – Experience cravings

This is the most important experiment. It will enlighten you on how sensitive you are to white carbohydrates. It will allow you to apply the Rule #1 and Rule #2 of the CogniDiet® Sugar Control Plan. I want you to feel for yourself what happens when you start the day with different breakfasts.

- **Day 1:** Have a high sugar breakfast. Start with one or two slices of white bread, bagel or croissant or muffin, with jam or honey, plus a fruit or a fruit juice (freshly squeezed or from a bottle). You could replace the toast with cereals and milk.
- **Day 2:** Have a source of protein such as an egg or two, or a slice of ham, tofu, or cheese with a slice of bread. You can add a fruit (no juices). Or have a cup of 1 to 2% fat yogurt (no sugar nor fruits added) with a real fruit, like berries.
- **Day 3:** Try a slow release good carbohydrate such as a half cup of cooked oatmeal with 1 to 2% fat dairy source (or other liquid such as water or almond milk). You can add an egg or a protein source. You could also try a half cup of breakfast chili, mixing beans/lentils with a protein.

Notice your energy, brain power and sugar cravings within the next hours. How long can you go without a need for more food? And what type of food?

The Day 1 breakfast is very high in fast releasing sugars. The other breakfasts are combining fat and protein, and slow release carbohydrates.

Experiment #2 – Become a label sleuth

Go to the grocery store or shop in your kitchen, and look at labels. Select cereals, ice creams, cookies, tomato sauce, frozen dinners, breads, breads, and yes dressings!

How many carbohydrates do you see on the label?

- What is a real serving? The calories announced are only per serving.

- Is there added sugar? Look at the list of ingredients. Some foods contain natural sugar, like lactose in milk or dairy, but they may also have extra sugar added.

- Do you see the difference between carbohydrates, sugar and fiber? It does not add up. Look at the label information below. I remember a client telling me she was a good girl because she bought a no sugar added muffin. She forgot to count flour as a source of glucose.

One 4 oz. muffin – Plain
No added chocolate chips, nuts, fruits, etc.

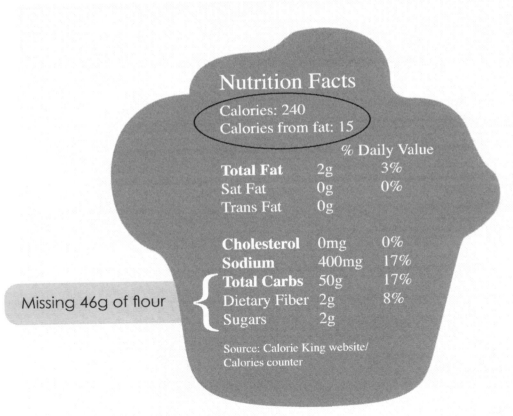

Nutrition Facts

Calories: 240
Calories from fat: 15

		% Daily Value
Total Fat	2g	3%
Sat Fat	0g	0%
Trans Fat	0g	
Cholesterol	0mg	0%
Sodium	400mg	17%
Total Carbs	50g	17%
Dietary Fiber	2g	8%
Sugars	2g	

Missing 46g of flour

Source: Calorie King website/
Calories counter

Experiment #3 – Know how many carbohydrates you eat

Assess how many carbohydrates you ate yesterday, or on a typical day, using the table below. Use one of the apps we recommend later in this chapter. Then for fun transform the grams (except non-starchy vegetables) in mountains of sugar.

To simplify the game, imagine that 4g of carbs = 4 grams of sugar = 1 teaspoon of sugar. Remember to count Net Carbs.

Meal – include alcohol and sugary drinks	Net Grams of Carbohydrates
Breakfast	
Lunch	
Dinner	
Snacks	
TOTAL teaspoons of sugar	Except for non-starchy vegetables, transform all carbohydrates in mountains of sugar.

What are your insights? Do you realize how quickly it accumulates? How much of these carbohydrates are really fresh vegetables? You should be eating at least 5 to 7 cups a day (cooked or uncooked). YES, you should!

Experiment #4 – Eliminate certain foods

Write a plan of action for SUGAR elimination. What are the foods you can eliminate or decide to substitute healthier options with?

- What is in your cabinets at home? Get rid of what you do not want anymore
- Create a stash of healthy snacks at your desk, at the office or where you know you are most vulnerable and most likely to go to the "vending machine"
- Make it a priority to find new healthier snacks that will replace older, more sugary or processed snacks

Go without any sugar, including fruits, for one day. Try to stick to vegetables and limited slow release carbohydrates such as oatmeal for breakfast. This is one step further than the breakfast experiment. Write down your craving level, feelings, emotions, energy level and mood. If you can try to continue for a few more days and again, write down how you feel. See how you transform.

Experiment #5 – Create your list of benefits being sugar-free

Create the list of all your personal benefits for eliminating sugar—this is the cognitive behavioral aspect of this program. The previous experiments should help you find out more about how you feel. Please write full sentences in your diary. And always start with the word "I." Examples:

- I do not have cheap ice cream buckets in my freezer anymore. It created a bad habit of splurging every night in front of the TV. I now treat myself to an excellent, locally made and organic ice cream once a week that I eat very mindfully
- I have "Feng shui-ed" my kitchen from all the sugar laden condiments, dressing and drinks. I feel liberated. I realized I got rid of 4,000g of sugar. I calculated that all these products together represented 1,000 teaspoons of sugar or 16,000 calories!
- I cut my sugar intake by 50% this week and I feel so much better. I lost 10 pounds, wow, this is how I feel now:
  - ✓ More energetic
  - ✓ Sharper
  - ✓ Less tired
  - ✓ Less puffy
  - ✓ I slept better

- ✓ More optimistic
- ✓ I walk faster and work longer hours
- ✓ I did not look for sweets every 2 hours as usual

- I have made a list of all the impact this sugar cutting has had on my health and I can't wait to see the new blood data:

  - ✓ I will lower my body fat
  - ✓ I will lower my blood pressure and cholesterol numbers
  - ✓ I will lower my risk for diabetes – I am borderline pre-diabetic

CogniDiet® Book Club Discussion Guide

This week you have plenty to do with the five experiments. I recommend that you perform all the experiments. It is crucial to do Experiment #1, because this will show you what sugar does to you.

The group members who really cut white and starchy carbs and sugar this week will have the most impressive weight loss results. If you have sophisticated scales, you may also be able to notice how much water you lost.

- **Discuss how you notice changes within your group (physical and energetic changes). It is always very good to hear compliments from or be inspired by your friends.**

- **How was Experiment #1?**

- **How did you feel this week after eliminating sugar and carbs? How did you feel on the first days?**

- **Cook with a carb substitute if you have dinner or lunch together**

- **What have you discovered about sugar in general?**

- **What have you learned with the experiments?**

- **If somebody keeps on finding excuses, push them to commit!**

You may now have a weight loss winner already! Or some of you need encouragement. Have a list of actions after the meeting.

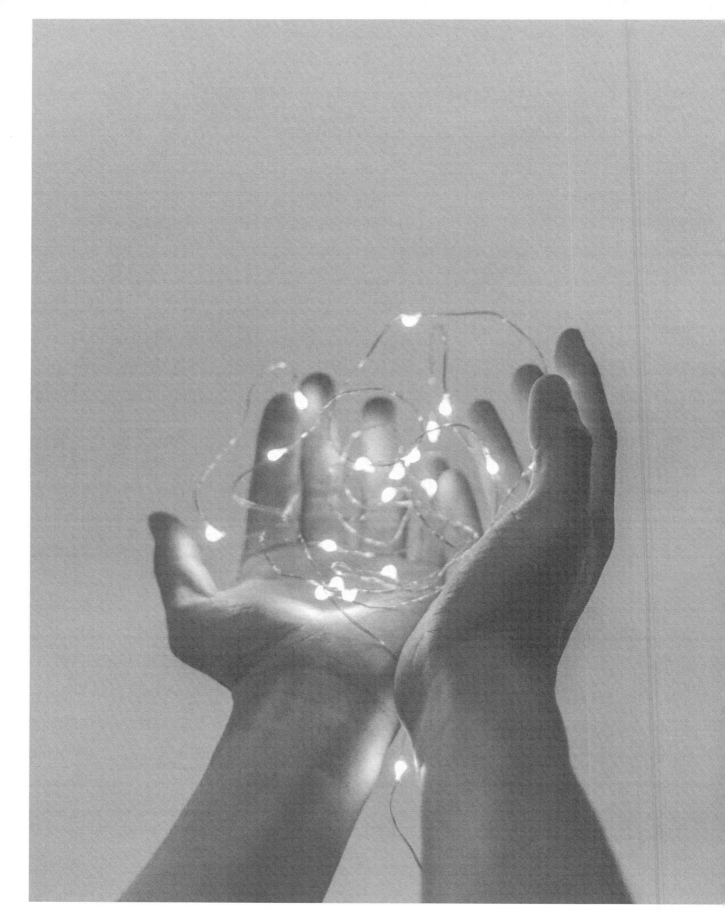

Chapter 3

I Am Rewiring My Brain

Nothing Beats the Pleasure of a Fresh Thought

Have you ever taken the time to retrace your steps and look at what you did on a day where you felt you went astray, or one where you just conducted business as usual? The unnecessary snack at 10 a.m., followed by the sugary coffee while shopping for food. And then, oh yes, the delicious pineapple upside down cake at lunch with a friend. Gosh another 500 calories, whipped cream not included. "Well, it's only today! I will get back on track tomorrow," you tell yourself.

But as you work on your computer doing your taxes in the afternoon, you mindlessly eat candied nuts out of a bag. They just happened to be in your drawer. Because you have snacks everywhere in the house and at the office. After dinner, as you watch TV with your family, you share pretzels with your husband, because this is your evening ritual. At this stage, you don't even know why you do this anymore, just because...

The next day you decide to be a good girl, which lasts until the afternoon when you attend a girlfriends' party with dangerously attractive appetizers and wine. Ah, the mini pizza bites, the pigs in a blanket, the one bite salmon quiche and the wine. Each bite is at least 30 to 40 calories, no kidding, but everybody is eating, so why not me!

You tell yourself: "I will start my diet on tomorrow." This is your permission cue. This is one of the most powerful sabotaging thoughts ever. This is the magic way to allow yourself to eat and drink whatever you wish this week. But then the next day comes and just another reason to not pay attention and an excuse to postpone the resolution again to the next day, or week. One week later you gained two pounds, darn it!

Here you are today. The pounds are packing on, you have been on multiple diets, and you all know them by name. You are an expert at finding what is new and hot. "Let me try the new Atkins. Paleo is so in now. Why not experience the HCG* miracle diet, Suzie lost 30 pounds in two months?"

On Facebook and Pinterest, you are so good at sharing new healthy recipes, cool food posts, and you follow all the diet and nutrition gurus. You have 30 diet books on your bookshelves at home as well. You know it all. And yet…

Now you are valiantly embarking on another diet. One of your girlfriends swears it is the best one yet. It requires you to spend $600 on organic and gluten free pre-packaged foods every month and you need to buy a three month supply. This is your third pre-packaged diet. The last two failed. But deep down you hope it will work this time, because it is organic – that is the subconscious new rationale! It is so much easier to embark on a new diet than really looking at yourself

---

*HCG is an acronym for human chorionic gonadotropin, a hormone produced by the placenta after implantation. This diet promotes the use of this hormone via injection or oral ingestion and is associated with a 500 calorie a day diet (!!) for 8 weeks.

and dealing with the root cause of your overeating. I am chuckling because I have done that. I remember a liquid diet, and the chemical shakes ended up, after one week, gathering dust in the garage! They were so disgusting and boring.

But this time you are motivated. The sugar is gone for three weeks and the pounds are leaving the fortress. You keep the weight off for six months, but then sugar is slowly and surely crawling back in your life. You regained what you lost plus 20%. How discouraging. You feel defeated. You feel like a failure. And to make things worse, every year it gets harder and your metabolism slows down. You lose approximately two to four percent of your metabolic strength each decade.

You are the constant dieter. Diet is like an annoying lover. You live, sleep, think, drink and eat with it day and night, maybe 150 days out of 365 a year. And this for the past 20 years. You can say with a good laugh and a tragic realization that you have been dieting for 3,000 days out of your otherwise awesome life. And you gained 40 pounds over the same period or two extra pounds a year. How frustrating.

Three thousand days wasted in not eating what you like, being grumpy and unsatisfied most of the time. Three thousand days of positive energy lost in shopping for special foods, spending fortunes on milkshakes and processed foods, depriving yourself of joy. Let's face it, who says "I am so happy to be on a diet?"

Cogni-Game:

Calculate. "For the past 10 to 20 years, I have been on a diet for _____ days."

And how do you feel when you "diet." What are the words that come to mind? Write them down. And reflect upon them. **Is it:**

- Hungry most of the time
- Unsatisfied
- Obsessed with foods I cannot eat
- Deprived
- Punished
- Unfair
- Starving
- Stressed out
- Angry etc.

Back to me. I was a constant dieter, especially when I started to live in the U.S. I gained 30 pounds coming here. Lose, gain, lose, gain, lose, and gain again. There came a time when I said to myself "it's over!"

Enough is enough. Stop finding excuses.

Enough is enough! Stop finding excuses. Stop saying "I'll try" or "I'll do my best." Let's commit to change today in this chapter. That happened to me in 2006. There was a trigger point. It was my health and my looks, but health was the primary reason. A new vision emerged, like a hope, a way out, a plan of escape. I did not create a vision board. I did not write new positive thoughts. I did not know what they were at that point. But I became more educated about what foods did to me. Remember, I went to nutrition school. Not that you all have to become nutritionists. But there is so much available information now that you can become more curious and courageous at facing your triggers and food issues. I hope today is your day.

I want to give you hope. I want to inspire you. I want you to know you are not alone. This book and program were written to help you. I hear you, sister. It is difficult to do it on your own. You may have lost motivation.

Did you do your homework in Chapter 1? Where is your vision board? Can you see it from here, as you read this page? I hope that by now you feel more energized again because of your new vision. If not, go back to that chapter immediately.

I will help you create new pathways in your brain and enjoy new behaviors that will set you free of the past and allow you to make your vision come true.

Cogni-Game:

Write this in your diary: "For the next 10 years I will eat naturally for most of the days in a year. I will get my 3,000 lost days back."

What I want you to say is "This is the way I will eat for the rest of my life!" I believe you can achieve this if you stick to an 80% attainment goal for CONTROL and leave 20% for the usual treat, unplanned event or moment of weakness.

Now, write how you would feel living a diet free life:

Are you:

- Inspired
- Free
- Lighter
- Enjoying life
- Happy
- Healthy
- Liberated etc.

This is my philosophy. Life is what it is. We all love sugar. We are conditioned to love sugar from the day we are born because it is contained in the maternal milk. We need carbohydrates as fuel. So let's be good 80% of the time. That is possible. This is feasible. Your brain will still be happy.

As I said earlier, your brain is a very mysterious animal. Its sinuous convolutions and compartments are still very "terra incognita" for the most parts. There is no real map for circulation in that upper room. Deep secrets are sleeping in your subconscious mind, very often sabotaging or even contradicting your stated desires. The logical mind gets high jacked by stress. The external world takes control over your life's direction and decisions.

I always say to my client that in order to get rid of dieting, you have to think differently. You have to forget about diets. You have to start to focus on yourself and your desire for change.

Cogni-Tip:

Willpower is not enough. To change you need to focus on what matters to you most! And create new happy circuits in your brain.

Something else needs to occur. Let me ask you this week, and for the future, to regularly observe yourself and raise your behavioral self-awareness. What a sentence! In simpler words, just become aware of your eating choices. What is going on in your mind when you start to think about having an ice cream?

This is where it starts. Instead of going through life like a robot—we all do it as the pace of life increases—just take a break with me. Hold my hand as you spend the day. And observe yourself. Stop in your tracks when you start to move your hand to open the fridge to seize the last brownie after a good dinner.

The power of your imagination and desire for transformation must become the beacons of your life. The desire to shed the weight and free yourself must be so strong and deep that the force and energy it breeds enables you to move mountains—of pretzels—out of your way.

The tipping point is when the pleasure your brain gets from being at your healthy weight and all the benefits it brings you (remember Chapter 1) including enjoying a delicious and nutritious arugula salad with fresh grapefruits, is stronger than the pleasure of shoving yet another candy in your mouth.

Cogni-Game:

When was it that you had a craving and yielded to it? Look at that treat with a magnifying glass. Write down what it is. Note the ingredients. Describe the pleasure, or not really, that you derived from it, before and after:

- Just looking at the wrapping makes me salivate

- Opening the wrapper and smelling the chocolate gets me all excited already

- It feels sweet and soft in my mouth, it melts in my throat and the flavor lingers on my palate

- One minute of pleasure

- I feel very happy for a few seconds, and then I want more. After six, I feel disgusted.

INSTANT Cogni-Shift:

Now, picture yourself at your ideal weight. Note the pleasure and satisfaction derived from being able to run again, or get to a smaller clothes size, feeling attractive, happy and energetic. Write the words to describe these emotions. And then close your eyes and feel these feelings as intensely as you can. Here are a few possible ones:

- I am surrounded by a cloud of positive energy
- People are attracted to me because I smile and they love my conversation
- I am feeling so pretty in my floral dress (it has been in my closet, too small, for 5 years)
- My best friend payed me the best compliment today
- My eyes are finally coming out. I felt the fat around them hid them!

You just started to create a new happy pathway in your brain. Light has flooded the room.

Now try to re-write these words using all your senses (smell, taste, sight, etc.). This will make all parts of your brain happy.

Examples for inspiration, create your own:

- **Sight:** "I look attractive in that dress." This thought illuminates your self-worth and self-esteem pathways. It chases away your old self-pity and negative views of yourself.

- **Smell:** "I walk in a garden after the rain, full of energy, I smell the roses and they remind me of my beautiful grandmother who was always working in the garden with me." This happy thought drives you back to a healthy childhood moment. Your grandmother was beautiful and inspired you to take care of yourself.

- **Taste:** "I enjoy eating these vegetables so much now. I can taste the earthy flavors, the powerful nutrients, and the exotic and pleasing spices used to cook them." This will make you really feel good about yourself.

- **Touch:** "I never looked at an artichoke this way. I peeled it and admired all the textures and colors. There is some purple even. It is soft inside but well-guarded."

At this point your brain is firing from all angles. All these pleasing words associating with the experience create new connections. New souvenirs linked with senses are created. They become stronger as you continue to change.

You unravel old knots, linked to other experiences that may not have been as healthy for you. And as you know, change is not happening overnight. It is the doing it every day that will help you get your brain to transform.

You have fast forwarded your energy into a new positive endeavor. But if you continue to prioritize the immediate pleasure derived from sipping a 500-calorie flavored coffee, over your vision, you will not lose weight. In this chapter we will give you the tools to find your own sabotaging thoughts, sometimes profoundly ingrained in your brain, and transform them into radiant, amazing, positive thoughts leading to new behaviors. We will help you transform old habits into newer, healthier ones that will support your blossoming into an amazing, awesome, terribly inspiring new YOU.

INSTANT Cogni-Shift:

> Imagine yourself as a rose blooming under the sun. Think about the process and how each layer of petals opens up one after the other. Synchronize with your breath. Inhale, open the petals, exhale and close the petals.

Describe how you feel and look in your vision board again. Think about your 5 senses:

I am radiant with positive warmth. Happiness is reflected in my eyes and smile. My skin is glowing because I feed it with so many good nutrients. My belly is flat again and soft to the touch. My hair is shiny and healthy, etc.

The SATs and PATs

Now, we are going to start to work on your positive amazing thoughts (remember we call them PATs). But before we do this, you will have to spend a few days observing yourself and discovering your biggest awful sabotaging thoughts or the SATs as we call them. Here below are a few that I have heard a lot over the years:

- I want to eat this now, it is just a bite, I'll exercise later today.
- I am traveling, it is impossible to be good. I will get back on track when I am back home.
- I had a tough meeting, I deserve that cookie.
- It's Halloween, Thanksgiving, etc. Why start my diet now?
- I cannot say no to a second helping, it would be rude to the hostess
- I paid for all this, I may as well eat it.
- Why start now at 60 years old? I failed for over 40 years, why would I succeed now?
- I can eat as much as I want as they say it is sugar free.
- I am fine, because it is organic and fresh!
- It is only a 100-calorie package...

SATs are your enemy. They sabotage your attempts, they misdirect your energy and they prevent you from adopting new behaviors. They have often been ingrained in your brain and subconscious for years. They may be there because of the way you were raised. Maybe you had a critical mother, or a not so nice sister. You may have been bullied at school.

What are yours? Maybe you need some time to realize what is going on. One of my clients said to me after one week playing brain detective: "I don't even know what is going on in my brain. I am totally not aware of my thoughts and the reasons why I look for chocolate. This is my big insight this week." It took her another week to finally realize that food was her reward for all the hard work she was putting into her career as a family breadwinner. Her life was empty, there was no love. She filled the vacuum with food. Her biggest SAT was: "I am suffering so much, I need one pleasure in my life, and I deserve it."

Cogni-Tip:

If you feel it's too hard to find what's going on in your brain, just stop one minute before you take that bite. The insight could appear at that moment or later in the day. It is important to find **PATTERNS.**

I believe my client's struggle to find out her SATs was because, deep inside, she did not want to know. At least initially. So to unstick her, I asked her to go directly to her PATs and become aware of her most challenging situations. So before I ask you to embark and find your SATs and replace them with PATs, you need to also realize what most situations they are associated with.

Most Frequent Sabotaging Situations

Everybody has a different life. And different challenges. Some situations are more often encountered than others. A tough one for me would be to work in the best pastry shop in the city. Smell and view of croissants and lemon tarts would still today drive me right to sugar hell.

I guess my advice here would be to find another job! Not easy you will say, but then you have to develop coping skills. And what about the person who travels constantly, and not to the most health conscious parts of the world. It is easy to find healthy food in New York City. But what about certain cities in the middle of nowhere where the only restaurants are fast food ones?

Maybe you spend so much time in your car. Or you are an at-home mother surrounded by loving saboteurs! What are your most common challenging situations, where you know, unwanted cravings will be triggered? They may be related to:

- Work
- Home/family
- Parties
- Travel
- Stress
- Boredom
- Emotions (happy or unhappy)
- Memories
- Ingrained habits or rituals
- Food cues – remember how powerful smell and vision are! This includes the vision of an ad on TV or a shop on the road etc.

find the pattern

Example #1: *"My biggest sabotaging situation is when I am under pressure. My thought is that I try to escape the work by taking a break. I go to have a pretzel in the kitchen. I deserve it because I suffer.*

The sugar in the pretzel gives me a very short respite and a mini dopamine boost. It only lasts 10 seconds.

My discovery is that the pretzel does not solve the deadline issue, only the growing waistline issue!"

Example #2: *"My biggest sabotaging situation is parties. I attend a lot of social events and honestly like food.*

My thought is that I must go with the flow like others and that I will be better tomorrow.

I get all the delicious, yet calorie laden foods on the buffet and drink wine. I don't even realize how much I am eating.

I fool myself by saying that these are mini-bites. At the end of the party I feel guilty and realize I only ate "bad" foods. My SAT is that I will go on a diet tomorrow.

My discovery is that I have zero control. I am like a robot. But maybe it is because I am socially shy and the eating gives me confidence."

Write your own most frequent challenges, and peel the layers about what is going on in your head. It may take a week or two to really find out what is going on.

_____

_____

_____

_____

_____

My Biggest SATs/Associate Them With a Situation

_____

_____

_____

_____

_____

Now that you have realized your most important SATs, we will focus on replacing them with PATs. And I will tell you why. SATs will always initially be stronger than PATs. The mental pathway of the PAT needs more repetition. It is fighting a 20 year old SAT!

- PATs are developed by you in light of your goals—remember Chapter 2, and in order to retrain your brain to annihilate a current SAT

- They help you think before a decision is made and go back to your rational brain and behavior

- They rewire your brain so that you focus on the future/victories and not on the past/failures anymore

- They are linked with your new vision (remember, how do you want to feel and look?)

- It is highly recommended you accompany this with ways to decrease your stress level especially just before a moment when you know there will be temptations around you.

PATs, as you exercise your brain, will create new behavioral pathways and influence your future decisions. They will replace SATs and build your NEW resistance to temptations. They will help you change over time and will require daily training discipline.

Cogni-Tip:

Rome was not built in one day. Agassi did not become a tennis champion in one week. Even Einstein had to work. If you don't practice, your brain won't change!

How to Build My New PATs

The Sabotaging Thought	The Positively Amazing Thought!
I will never lose weight, I am too old and I have failed for 20 years.	I have the power and the tools to change. Let's do it. Trying something different never hurts.
I will start on Monday, to heck with paying attention this weekend. It is Memorial Day, let's have fun.	My calorie needs are the same on weekends and weekdays. I can enjoy myself while staying in control. I have my "calorie budget" this weekend and it allows me for a dessert on Sunday. So I can have fun, enjoy the company and still have my treat.
I cannot say 'NO" to a second helping, it will hurt the hostess' feelings.	Why lose the success of my past 5 days in one dinner? After all it is my body, my appetite. I can deal with saying "NO" in a gracious way.
I feel stuffed but I want more of these amazing pasta marinara, it's so delicious. I may never eat this again.	This is enough now, I enjoyed it. I can always come back to this restaurant or ask for and reproduce the recipe. And tomorrow I may have another amazing experience.
I deserve this chocolate cookie. I am miserable. I suffered enough today.	Well, how will I feel after the cookie? This is not going to solve the issue at hand.

You can also build your PATs as they relate to other issues in your life. For instance, you may be sabotaging your exercise efforts, or your desire to have less clutter in your house. We recommend you start to recognize your most sabotaging thoughts and then replace them with a positive statement.

Cogni-Tip:

The PAT is not enough. The new positively amazing thought has to lead to **A NEW ACTION** or **BEHAVIOR**. You cannot eat the cookie while thinking about a reason you should not! Find a distraction strategy.

· ·

This Week's Experiments

Experiment #1: Create your new PATs

Create your grid with your most common SATs and PATs and try to also see a pattern. Is this linked to specific situations? **Try to focus on your top 5.**

My Sabotaging Awful Thoughts/ Situations	My Positively Amazing Thoughts

What are you learning from this? Remember you have to add an ACTION to help your PAT create a new behavior, therefore pathway in your brain.

Create your list of ACTIONS. This experiment is about finding out what are your absolute worst craving triggering situations. For me at one point, it was to enter a Dunkin Donut®, because the view of the doughnuts initiated an irrepressible desire to have one. Then the whole morning unraveled and the sugar in the doughnut started a cycle of new cravings.

I realized I had to stop going there. Now by the way, I can go there, and I will not buy a doughnut anymore. I know their ingredients too well!

Instead, now, I go to another coffee shop or I bring a cup in my car with home brewed coffee. This is my new ACTION. My new PAT is: "I do not need these doughnuts. They do not nourish me and trigger an uncontrolled cycle of sugar craving. My coffee is enough to make me happy going to work. I just had breakfast!"

Experiment #2: Describe your new favorite healthy foods

Create a list of your new favorite, healthy foods. Now, associate each of them with positive words. Write these feelings and descriptions on paper. This will reinforce the experiment's value and convert new pleasure pathways in lasting memories.

Example: I just discovered I like eggplants and I learned to cook them in many different ways. How can I describe what I like about them? You could say:

- I like the beautiful, shiny skin and purple color of this vegetable
- I like the smell and taste of the eggplant especially when it has that burnt aroma
- I like the eggplant in a puree with garlic as it has this very unctuous texture
- It feels so smooth and creamy in my throat. I feel it is a God given gift from nature

Maybe you discovered you love kefir, a fermented and probiotic rich yogurt? Or maybe you just started to eat more fish and discover new ones like cod, skate, lemon sole, etc. Find a few new favorite healthy foods. The more you involve all your senses in an experiment, the more different parts of your brain get "illuminated" and help you change. The choice of specific words will elicit different responses. As an example the word "silky" will make you fire neurons in the brain touch-sensory area.

Take pictures of foods you love, healthy meals you love and take the habit of looking at them. Maybe put pictures in your diary or scrap book.

Experiment #3: Stand up for yourself at a party, or any gathering, even a family meal

You are at a restaurant with a group or at a party. It has to be an environment where you are not really in control of what is happening. You have to go with the flow while trying to stay in control.

Decide in advance (you can almost always see menus on line) or at the moment when you see the buffet or the menu about what you will eat and what you will drink.

Eat and drink slowly, especially if you are surrounded by big eaters or drinkers. Don't tell anybody you are doing the experiment but be conscious of what you put in your mouth. Enjoy the company and focus on the conversation, not what is in everybody's plate.

If they ask you to share a dessert, or want to pour you wine, prepare to say NO in a very polite yet firm manner. What can you say?

- Thank you, I had enough
- I am full, no room left
- I am not hungry anymore, really
- No drinking tonight, I am driving

Find your way of saying "no" in a nice way. How are others reacting?

- Are they teasing you?
- Are they or not paying attention to what/how you eat?
- Are they too busy enjoying themselves?
- Are they pushing you with remarks such as "ah, Emma is on a diet again?" or "party pooper, why can't you enjoy yourself, you can go on a diet tomorrow?"

What are you doing to stand up for yourself? Prepare your strategy next time you go out and you will be surprised to find out that a) people do not pay as much attention as you think to what you eat or drink and b) it is easier than believed to say NO politely, but firmly. Also pushing you to eat or drink, and share a dessert for instance, is their own way to give themselves permission to indulge – their SAT! They find an accomplice, so they take away half of their guilt.

Experiment #4: Be in control of your food

Write down your menu for the week and prepare your foods in advance, if you can. Bring your own food to work if you are based in an office. Or bring your own healthy choices to parties, as a gift, so at least you can stay semi in charge by eating what YOU want. You will be surprised at how many people will enjoy your healthy plate!

You do not have to do this perfectly. I do not want you to stress out. But apply the 80/20 rule. Be good in 80% of the situations. Even 70% is good enough when you start.

After the day or the party, write down the list of your insights and victories:

- What have you learned about yourself and others?
- Who is supporting you and who is sabotaging you?
- What were you able to control – like removing the cookie platter from the middle of the table?
- Maybe it is time to take some extra measures with your home or office environment – like the bowls of sweets on your desk?
- Maybe it is a good idea to stop going to lunch with Maria, because she always wants to go to rather unhealthy restaurants. Or maybe it is time to avoid the office kitchen for lunch because there is always cake and unhealthy foods tempting you there.

Experiment #5: Observe your fellow humans eating or shopping for foods

Just enjoy a day and walk in a city or in a shopping mall. Observe the multiple shops and stands where people can buy food or drinks. Become aware of the incredible multitude of opportunities we are being offered to buy something.

Are the food shops mostly healthy or unhealthy? Where do you see most people going? Just imagine you are writing a report about your observations.

Observe people walking with something to eat or drink in their hands. How do they eat while walking? On the same or another day, observe people eating in a restaurant or at a fast food place. How long does it take them to eat? How are they eating? How are they seated (are they even seated)? Look at their choices and portions. Look at their waist size, their personality etc. Be discreet however! You do not want to look like you are spying on them.

Your homework is to select a few persons. Observe them, and then write their imaginary eating and general life style habits. How do you correlate the supposed lifestyle with the physical appearance and observed eating behavior? By understanding your fellow humans, you may find out a few things about yourself too. For instance, very revealing will be the person you select.

I recommend you select somebody who would be a role model and somebody who would not. At the end of your report, meditate on what you learned, including some possible preconceived notions.

This concludes this chapter which is a very important one again for getting at the root of your challenges. The CogniDiet® philosophy is that the more you focus on what you can do and what you enjoy, the happier you are.

If you only like fast food and sugar but you are reading this book, it means you want to change the way you eat. There is always a way when there is a will. There are so many healthy foods that I cannot believe you would not find a couple that would satisfy you and re-design your palate for new tastes and textures, while filling you with vibrant nutrients. This is what happened to Debra. She really changed and as I write this page, she must be approaching 70 pounds lost!

Debra's Story: Adopting New Behaviors

Debra is a wonderful lady who did my clinical trial and became our biggest loser. She lost 33 pounds in 12 weeks and by December 2017, or 12 months after the trial, she had lost 80 pounds. Let me tell you that she looks 10 years younger. She had a habit of eating mostly processed and sugary foods. "Eating healthy, cutting out sugar, processed foods and carbohydrates that are nutrient poor is not a new idea. So why is this time different for me? Why did THIS program work?" asks Debra.

"First, my motivation for starting the CogniDiet®, was not to "look better." It was to avoid becoming diabetic, a disease my mother and brother struggle to manage. "

Her eternal sabotaging thoughts were:

- I love bread, I can't give it up
- I don't want to give up sweets, that's my reward.

They became:

- I need to learn how to manage these cravings or I will become diabetic like my family.

She learned to stop "eating her emotions." Sugar and carbs became less attractive and cravings diminished. Before, she would buy a pint of ice cream and eat it in one evening, always had cookies or cake in the house, and breakfast was coffee and a bagel or doughnut.

Her new behaviors:

- No sweets or white carbohydrates in the house.
- Keeping hard boiled eggs or oatmeal at hand for "on the go" breakfasts.
- Cake or ice cream are only for special occasions.

"A big "Aha" moment for me was doing my taxes after completing the clinical trial. In December 2016. When I was looking over receipts, I realized that prior to the CogniDiet®, every time I went into a store I was buying something sugary to eat. I was shocked. I had no idea I was in such a destructive pattern," she said.

Now, instead of constantly buying sugary treats, she purchases good quality products, experiment with cooking new things that are delicious and healthy, and plans her meals. Mindless, emotional and stress eating were her safety net. "Learning to be mindful included really looking and seeing my physical self, something I'd avoided," she says. The CogniDiet® also slimmed down her closet. She had held onto clothes in several different sizes, either in the hopes of getting back into them or in case she gained weight. "There is great freedom in not having closets that are packed with stuff that doesn't fit. It makes room for all types of new things that have nothing to do with clothes," she said. Debra has a new career, a new life and has completely re-invented herself in the process of losing weight.

CogniDiet® Book Club Discussion Guide

This week it's all about your old SATs, new PATs and behaviors. Observing yourself and others eating is an enlightening experience! I hope you have been good at capturing your thoughts in your diary. Writing, repeating, persisting is the way you will rewire your brain.

- **Share your new PATs, challenges and successes this week**

- **Have you discovered new healthy foods and recipes you like?**

- **Have you been in situations where you had to say "No, thank you"?**

- **What have you learned from observing other people?**

- **What are your goals for next week?**

- **How do you feel about yourself right now?**

Maybe it is time to plan a group outing in a "dangerous" restaurant? Navigate temptations together and choose a healthy meal. See how much fun you can have without a Pina colada and a chocolate cake!

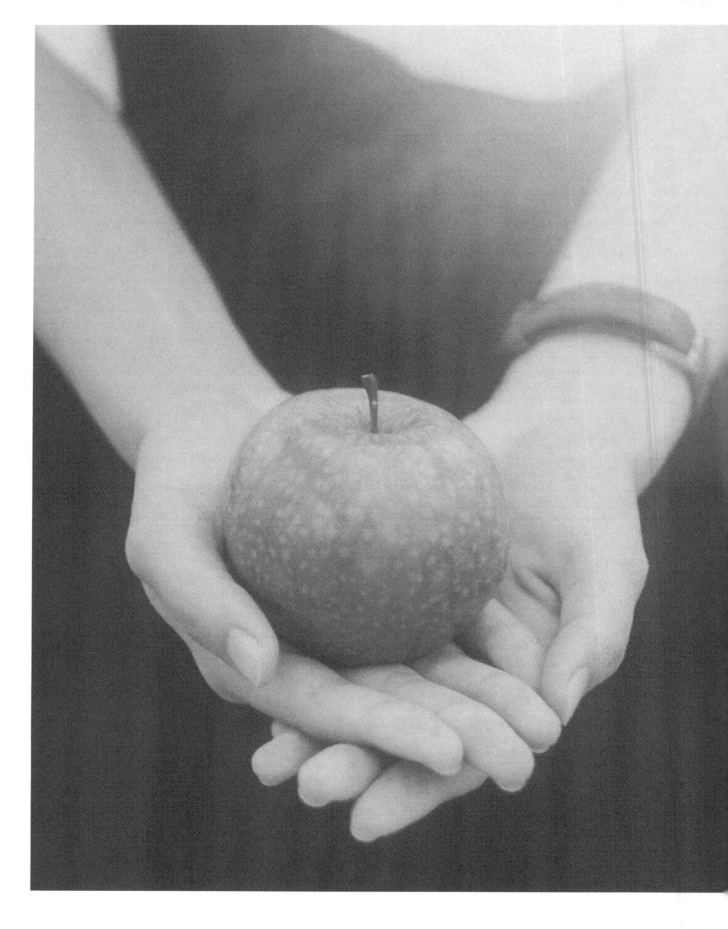

Chapter 4

My Body is a Temple...With Limited Square Feet

You Become What You Eat

By now you have learned to limit your sugar intake, create new healthy behaviors with your goals and create a vision of your future self as your inspiration. You have discovered many of your sabotaging behaviors and unhealthy eating patterns. By this time in the 12-week program, and especially if you cut the sugar and white carbohydrates, you must be managing your cravings much more effectively and feel more in control. So far, the only part of the program in which we have talked about food was the chapter about sugar. We have not covered fat nor protein. The reason is that I want you to focus on yourself and your behaviors.

You must have lost five to 10 pounds, if not more. Remember that sugar elimination (including processed foods that are laden with sugar) has enabled most of my clients to lose 10 to 15 pounds in the first week. It is always a great jumpstart and a "feel good" kind of achievement.

But you need to stay the course. The challenge after five to six weeks is to stay motivated and disciplined. Motivation is not enough unfortunately, and is not possible every day. Discipline and keeping your eyes on the goal is what will help you continue the transformation.

Here is a recap of what you need to do to continue meeting your weight loss goals.

The 8 CogniDiet® Principles You Need to Apply:

1. Excess sugar and carbohydrates (except non-starchy vegetables), including fruits, are the most important reason you are creating fat in your body. Continue to cut them out. Avoid them at dinner.

2. Always combine a protein and a fat with your carbohydrates (except non-starchy vegetables) to avoid future sugar/carbs cravings

3. Visualize your new YOU and your goals every day to stay the course

4. Recognize and apply your PATs and new actions every day

5. Write down and celebrate each one of your victories. Even the small ones — and they do not have to be related to the scales! You will not change overnight. But if you have a tough day get back in the saddle as soon as possible

6. Play the experiments, mind shifts and games. You can go back and play them again as many times as you want

7. The more you apply the CogniDiet® principles, the quicker your brain will change

8. Stay positive and enjoy life!

By now you are expecting a little bit more guidance. In this chapter, I will teach you about yet another myth. How much we need to eat every day. Life and working at The CogniDiet® has taught me that we eat way too much.

One of the biggest expressions of frustration I hear all the time — when participants have stopped losing weight after a while is:

- I am eating healthier
- I cut sugar
- I am eating whole carbohydrates instead of white ones
- I stopped snacking so much
- I eat and drink less in general
- I exercise more, etc.

There may be a few reasons you are stuck or not losing weight anymore, besides a possible real health issue like a lazy thyroid or mounting insulin resistance — which makes it even tougher to lose weight.

Maybe you are cheating. And you do not even realize it, yet. Or you are not just pushing yourself really outside a certain comfort zone. And I know why! We eat too much and in our society of overabundance, we do not even realize it anymore.

Here at the top seven reasons why you may not be losing weight:

1. You switch to healthy foods from unhealthier ones, but you still eat too many calories. A good example is adding too many nuts and cheese, which brings a lot of calories because of their fat content

2. You are cheating, and you don't tell. A little chocolate here, a glass of wine there. And before you know it, you accumulated an extra 500 calories in a day

3. You don't eat enough protein and good fat and still too many carbohydrates – even if whole, therefore healthier – such as oatmeal, whole grains, whole rice, whole bread etc.

4. You eat too many fruits and dairy. This equal sugar (fructose in fruits, lactose in dairy)

5. You still eat too much processed food which equals hidden sugar, bad fats and salt

6. You have not cut your portion size enough!

7. You exercise more, but as a consequence, you allow yourself to eat more as a reward. Remember that running for one hour at a reasonable pace may only burn 400-500 calories, which are contained in just one protein bar (200 to 300 calories) and one extra cookie (200 calories minimum).

Cogni-Game:

Write down, right now, the list of your cheats and rapidly try to estimate how many calories they represent. Do this on a regular base if you are frustrated with slow or lack of weight loss.

In this chapter we will help you understand how much you must eat to meet your daily physiological needs while losing weight, and in what ideal proportions. And yes, how you combine foods has an impact on your metabolism and can help you lose weight faster. We are moving from the detective and self-observation role to a more calorie-focused mindset.

After all, if you continue to eat too many calories, and of the wrong sort, you will not lose or continue to lose weight.

I am also a big believer that if you focus on what you can eat rather than what you cannot eat, it gives a positive perspective to your weight loss journey. You will learn about your metabolic basal rate (MBR) which gives you the calories you need every day as a minimum to survive.

The Basal Metabolic Rate or BMR

The basal metabolic rate, or BMR, is what you need to eat every day to help your body function and survive. You need calories and good nutrients to get your heart beating, your hair to grow, your digestion to occur. Every movement requires energy that is provided by burning fat.

When you look at standard tables, because they exist, they take into account age, sex and height. It will make sense that the bigger you are the more calories you need to function. And the more muscular you are the more calories you will burn, too, because muscles burn more calories than fat.

This is the formula. The BMR was established taking into account a minimum of activity. You need to add some extra fuel if you are exercising. Here is the table.

How to Calculate Your Calories

Basal Metabolic Rate (BMR) is the number of calories you would burn with NO activity

MEN

BMR + 66 + (6.23 x weight in lbs) + (12.7 x height in inches) - (6.8 x age)

Women

BMR + 655 + (4.34 x weight in lbs) + (4.7 x height in inches) - 4.7 x age

Your Target Daily Calorie Needs

1. Little or no exercise: BMR x 1.2
2. Light exercise/sports 103 days per week: BMR x 1.375
3. Medium Exercise/sports 3-5 days a week: BMR x 1.725
4. Intense exercise/sports, physical job or twice a day training: BMR x 1.9

Most women I have seen in my practice oscillate between 1,000 and 1,400 calories as a basic BMR. This is also what shows up on my professional body composition Rice Scale.

Calculate your base BMR. Here is the magic formula for women

655 + (4.35 X weight in pounds) + (4.7 X height in inches)

– (4.7 X age in years) = _____

Convention also stipulates that in general — again you may have a different metabolism — you need to burn an extra 2,000 (younger and more muscular women) to 3,500 calories a week, or 500 calories a day to lose ONE POUND a week. You could see results at 300 calories, some of you may go further. It all depends on different factors:

- Your core metabolism. The more you have been on restrictive diets, the more it is difficult to lose weight
- Your muscle mass. You could be a skinny fat lady!
- Your age
- Maybe a slow thyroid
- A very high sensitivity to carbohydrates or pre-diabetes

Let's say your base BMR is 1,200 calories. What is your caloric intake, on the days you exercise, and on the days you don't exercise?:

My Base BMR	I don't exercise at all	I exercise lightly
Example: 1,200 calories	1,200 X 1.2 = 1,440	1,200 X 1.375 = 1,650
I cut 300-500 calories a day for weight loss	1,200 calories (not recommended to go under 1,200 a day however, see how you are doing)	1,150-1,350 calories
Insert your numbers: _____ calories	_____	_____
Now cut 300-500 calories a day _____ calories	_____	_____

We often believe, when we go on a diet, that when we have lost the weight we want we can go back to the way we ate before the diet. For instance, you cut your calories to 1,200 a day when you were in fact eating 2,000 a day without exercising and gaining 12 pounds a year. Once you have lost the desired pounds, if you go back to the way you were eating, the pounds will come back, even more because you starved yourself. I know of women who cut their calories to 500 a day.

NO, NO, NO! And NO Again!

You do not need more that 1,400 to 1,600 calories to maintain your weight if your BMR is 1,200. And you will realize very quickly that this is just a formula.

You need to do some experiments to find out what it is that you need to eat:

- To lose weight, one to two pounds a week, no more, or
- To maintain your weight loss

Besides, you will also learn that food combinations will determine how you lose weight and maintain. 1,200 calories of just carbohydrates will, unless you are extremely young and active, make you gain weight! Remember insulin is a fat storing hormone. A combination of carbohydrates, good fat and protein will help you lose weight.

Portion Size and Combinations

In this chapter I want you to learn to evaluate your calories and portions at the glance of an eye. This is, based on my experience over 10 years of teaching healthy nutrition, the best and easiest way to manage your calories. Here are general recommendations but again they vary. Diet gurus and nutritionists all have their recommendations. It depends if you are on a high protein diet, a low carbs high fat diet (all the rage now), etc. Thousands of books have been written and stories shared: "I lost my fat with the cabbage soup diet," "I swear by the non-dairy, carb free and high fat regimen" and more...

The RDA recommends the 3/1/1 ratio which will read as this, for a diet of approximately 1,500 to 2,000 calories a day:

- 45 to 60% of carbohydrates (mostly vegetables and fruits, whole grain and legumes etc.)
- 20 to 30% of fat (mostly unsaturated fat and 10% max from saturated fat)
- 20 to 35% of proteins (preferably lean proteins)

This is a tricky part of the chapter. Remember, I said in Chapter 2 that to really lose and keep weight off you should limit your carbohydrates (except non-starchy vegetables) to 100 to 150mg a day, which represents 400 to 600 calories. If you are sticking to a 1,200 calorie a day diet to lose weight, this only leaves you with 800 to 600 calories for protein and fat.

If you are already insulin sensitive or borderline diabetic, you really, really need to watch your carbohydrates. I know that I need to watch for this like a hawk, to the point that I know I do not do well with beans and legumes. You may be different, and have no problems. You need to find out what works for you. Genes can have an impact as well. I just did my genotyping with a company I work with, Nutrigenomix®, and realized, after they mapped 45 of my nutritional genes that I had to be careful with grains and was slightly sensitive to gluten. I can gain two to three pounds overnight if I go for desserts, wine and bread at dinner! Of course it is mainly water. But still!

Again, you need to find out what works best for you within these parameters:

My needs	Percentage and total calories
Carbohydrates • Starchy • Other • Fruits (not more than 2 a day)	Is it 45 or 60%? _____
Protein	You will learn in a later chapter that women need an average of 50-60g a day
Fat – preferably non saturated and no trans fats	

INSTANT Cogni-Shift:

Visualize a healthy plate regularly before you eat. Become good at estimating what is in your plate in terms of calories. It does not have to be perfect.

Let's now explore how a client of mine downsized her portions and lost 20 pounds after having a baby. She realized also that it was all the little cheats here and there that were preventing her from reaching her goals.

Katia's Story – The Value of Cutting Portions

Katia (not her real name) is a young mother. One of my youngest clients. Life had been completely transformed with the baby and Katia was carrying extra weight after the pregnancy. She also worked. She initially struggled on the program, not taking the time really to focus on herself. What a surprise, yet another woman who puts everybody else ahead of herself.

I had a hard time finding out why she was not losing weight. Then she admitted she was munching a lot, left and right, as she said. Anything was good enough: cookies, sugary coffees, candies, potato chips, whatever. She was the type of woman who always wanted to taste what is in your plate, or have a bite of your dessert. She usually skipped lunch and was starving by the end of the day. There was wine at dinner, a good way to relax after a hard day.

She also realized, when we did the portion experiment that she was eating too much. Way too much: 1,000 extra calories. She did not count the "mini bites." She was also not exercising. She finally took a few measures, after almost six weeks of frustration and no weight loss, determined to make progress. At that stage she was very upset with herself. I told her that some people were slower than others to lose weight. That encouraged her without beating herself again.

Do not compare yourself to others. Everybody is different!

She had a hard time balancing her life between the baby, the husband, the job and the commute. Sound familiar? She took the bull by the horn and we designed an action plan. She did the following:

- She started to eat dinner on a dessert plate and in small bowls. She realized that in spite of having cut her portions, she was not hungry! She became more attuned to her real appetite. She started to lose one to two pounds a week.

- She stopped drinking any wine at dinner, not that she was drinking it often

- She brought lunch to the office (requires planning)

- She kept a diary. She became very disciplined about it and counted every morsel, and every bite she put in her mouth. She got a huge surprise. She realized she was regularly adding 300 to 400 calories to her daily diet and her BMR was 1,400 calories

- To avoid the extra little bites, because she liked to taste things, she did something silly but effective. She wrote **"no need"** on her hand along her thumb. It was discreet but each time she brought something to her mouth mindlessly she saw the words. She did this for two weeks. She lost three pounds.

- She however, allowed herself to have two very specific snacks at 10 a.m. and 4 p.m.. They were planned and always available.

- Once she tackled munching and her portion size she embarked on exercise. She bought an at home bike so she did not have to go to the gym and leave her baby for too long. She was using leaving the house as a SAT.

It's a short story but she credited her success to discovering what her real needs were and by abiding to a disciplined diary writing and snacking routine. She realized she was eating almost 2,000 to 2,500 calories a day. She had never had the guts to really measure what she was eating before. She did not want to know.

She finally faced the truth and the reality of her true needs. Now let's go to our experiments!

....

This Week's Experiments

Experiment #1: Learn to visualize your calories

Get an 9-10 inches diameter plate—that was your grandmother's china plate size—or try at least to not exceed 11 inches, and prepare a meal comprised of vegetables (not salads), a whole carbohydrate (quinoa, whole rice, sweet potatoes etc.), and 3 to 4oz. of meat/fish/poultry or a vegetarian option like tofu.

For vegetarians, I know the protein source is mostly soy based, beans and legumes. Some allow dairy which is a great source, or even eggs. There are so many differences between vegan, vegetarian, flexitarian, and other nuances. But again, at the end of the day, I have noticed a serious lack of protein and too many carbohydrates in my vegetarian clients.

They often come to see me with elevated glucose levels and are borderline diabetic or diabetics. My best advice in these instance is to look at adding protein powder to the diet, even if not ideal. There are many plant based protein available now with hemp, peas, nuts, etc. Remember what I said earlier in food combinations. You may have to start integrating more pure protein in your diet.

Experiment #2: Learn to work with a calorie counter for at least one week

I know I know, it is not fun to count calories and it is not a big part of my philosophy. However, you need to become aware of what you are putting in your body. Especially if at that stage you are not losing weight or are feeling stalled. I recommend MyFitnessPal®, a free app. In addition to counting calories, it allows you to track exercise and subtract it from your total. I also like the fact you can set your target macronutrient goals.

This is the one I use and recommend to my clients. There are other excellent apps such as:

- Lose It!®
- Spark People®
- Fat Secret®

There is always a new one, find the one you prefer

There are many others but at the end you have to select what works best for you. They all have their pros and cons. But I believe MyFitnessPal® is the easiest free app so far to use and gives enough information without having to buy the premium app. Do this for at least seven days and see how it influences your weight. Enter the data as soon as possible every day. Be creative when it comes to foods. Not everything is in the app database but you can take some shortcuts. When I have a salad I don't know what the exact dressing content is, but I add a tablespoon or two of oil as a surrogate. Or when I have a mixed salad I may enter the wrong vegetables but I know one cup of mixed salad is usually 25-30 calories, so I adjust the servings.

Cogni-Tip:

You do not need to get obsessive with calorie counting, but you must use this as a benchmark to see how it impacts your weight, up or down. And it is not only the calories that count, but the proportions between carbohydrates, protein and fat.

Experiment #3: The scale game. Understand the impact of certain foods on your weight

This game will throw you a little bit out of your comfort zone. It may even set you back as far as weight loss is concerned. But you need to be aware of what certain foods do to you. And also that your body undergoes mysterious changes that no amount or type of food or diet can explain. For instance, it took me a while to understand that getting my protein from beans and legumes did not sit well with me. I was eating too many carbohydrates. It is only when I eliminated them, replaced them with animal based protein, except for a few beans once in a while in salads etc., that I started to lose weight again.

- One night, when you go to a restaurant, or have a good dinner at home, include carbohydrates such as wine, bread/rice/fries etc. and even a dessert. You do not have to eat everything, just be a little bit more permissive with carbs. See the influence on the scale not only the next day but the next three days.
- For a few nights in a row only have non starchy vegetables and a protein at night. Again look at your scales the next days.

In this experiment, I want you to understand that excess is OK, we have a life, but the biggest sabotaging moment usually is that the weight gain or weight loss can take 2 to 3 days before it shows up. So people enjoy a pretty calorie-heavy dinner, don't see anything bad on the scale the next day and as consequence feel permission to continue to eat freely. Then the shock comes after a few days.

There is an almost contradictory advice I give my clients about the scales. Again, it is up to you. You need to stay in control. So maybe you like to do it every day. I believe that at the beginning of this program, you should do it often to understand how different foods may impact your weight. After that I suggest you go at least once a week, always at the same time of the day. And keep a diary!

Experiment #4: Deconstruct a sandwich, a pizza, a hamburger with fries

This one is an eye opener. I am inviting you to either really eat one of these or look online for their composition, using for instance your calorie counter app or getting the information from the company that is selling this food.

Having the food in front of you however is very different and more powerful from a "teachable moment" point of view that just doing it virtually. I have nothing against these foods but they are not what I would recommend as a staple in your diet.

Now deconstruct the food. See how it fits the 50% vegetables, 25% protein, and 25% starchy carbohydrates plate rule. After it's done, and you may have eaten it, reflect on the balance, the nourishment factor, the amount of calories and carbohydrates this meal presented.

Experiment #5: Each bite matters

This one will help you become more aware that what really sabotages a weight loss effort is not so much the rich and copious, once in a while, heavy meal or drinks. It is the everyday extra mini bites as I call them. I have a friend who is a specialist. She will be at the restaurant with me and try everything I eat. All in all, she must add 6-8 extra bites to her meal.

Each extra bite is 30 to 100 calories. Here are a few example. They are really approximations but I have realized that they are extremely useful at changing behaviors:

- A bite of cake or any pastry is usually around 30 calories but can creep up to 50 calories if it is a big bite of a decadent cake!

- A bite of finger foods, usually when you swallow the entire mini pizza or pig in a blanket at a party, is up to a whopping 100 calories.

- A mini wrapped portion of chocolate is usually 30 calories.

- A mini bite of vegetables dipped in dressing or hummus can be 50-100 calories, because of the fat contained in the dressing. Remember one tablespoon of any fat is usually 100 calories.

- Sampling foods in shops. Oh boy, this one is so dangerous!

- How many times in a day do you sample what you are cooking, finish your kids' plates, lick the remaining cake batter (who hasn't' done that, lol!). I estimate each extra bite can be 30 calories as well.

Before you bring this mini free bite to your mouth, stop, think about this experiment and make a decision. Do you really need to sample this? Why are you putting this in your mouth? What is the driver behind having a piece of cake with marmalade at Williams Sonoma® at 10 a.m., or cheese on cracker at Shoprite® at 7 p.m.? Do you really not know how it tastes?

CogniDiet® Book Club Discussion Guide

This week was all about becoming more attuned to your body's needs. Participants are always surprised to realize how much they eat versus how much they need. Our society has made a great effort at overblowing everything we eat and not only what is on our plate, but also sandwich, coffee, ice cream sizes. Cut them in half and usually it is still too much.

- **What is your no-exercise BMR? What is it when you add extra activities. Discuss.**

- **Are you using your calorie and macro counter or are you visualizing? Maybe the calorie counter is too complicated? Let's have somebody who knows it well explain to the others how to start and use it. This could be a whole session!**

- **Have you cut some calories this week? And if so, have you noticed results?**

- **What did you learn from deconstructing a sandwich or a pizza?**

- **What about the mini bites? Have you realized you had more of them than you thought?**

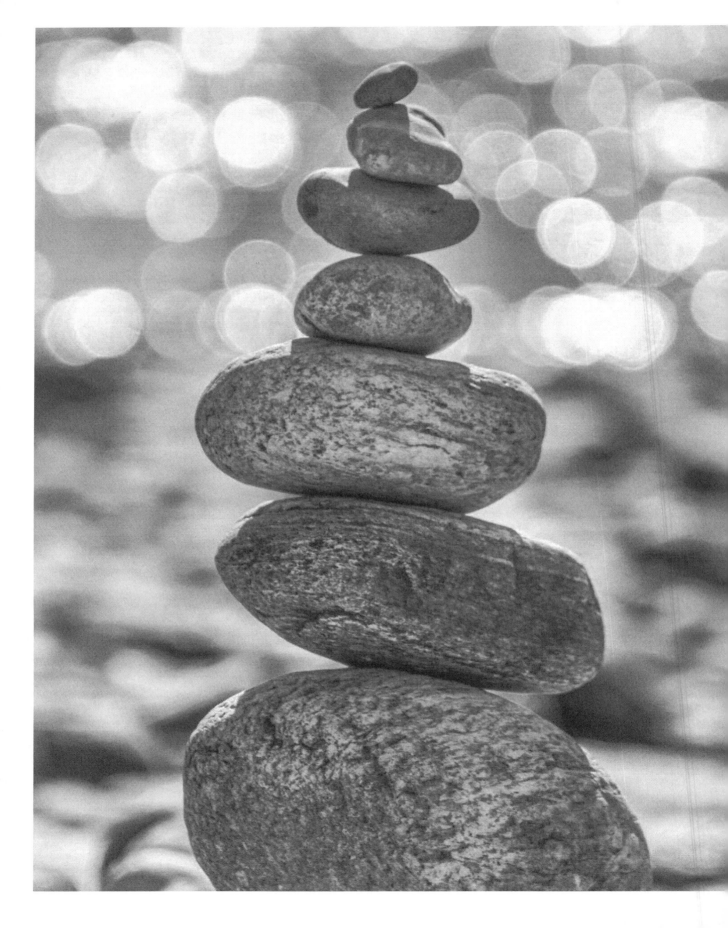

Chapter 5

Help, Stress Makes Me Fat!

Stress is the Biggest Saboteur

Stress almost killed me; I said it earlier. I have mixed feelings about this part of my life. On the one hand, I feel I should not have let myself go so low. On the other hand I had big financial obligations towards my family. But is financial obligation a good enough excuse, or the only excuse, to literally almost kill yourself at work? I was a highly paid executive. I could have chosen to downsize the house, the cars, the vacation, the shopping. I could have taken a paycheck cut or a job with less responsibilities. But I didn't. Not immediately.

There are many things I could have done differently to abate the stress level. Eventually I did, but I had to reach the bottom first. I was a slow learner. I am surprised how long I was able to go before I crashed.

And what am I complaining about? If you have a tough and not so well paying job, are hit with divorce and your kids have problems, there is no escape, there is no "downsizing" from life. There is no option to go to a lower paying job, because you are there already. You have to keep on going and meet your obligations. There is not often the luxury of options at that moment. You have to face reality and deal with your situation. My mother, who had a tough life, once said to me, as her third husband went bankrupt and she lost everything: "I do not have the luxury to get depressed, I have no time for that."

Some of us are born with a huge resilience factor—and my mother is an excellent example. She is an unshakable warrior with an amazing ability to find solutions in any situations and rebound from tragedy. Some of us are carried by faith or love. But some of us are more fragile or less resourceful. Some of us will break sooner than others. It does not have to be panic attacks, depression or burn-out symptoms. At least not initially.

Stress will sneak in your body and mind and attack all your organs, slowly but surely, day after day. Cancer may strike, a heart attack may hit or an ulcer may develop. I know it is not easy. I have met desperation and profound unhappiness in my clients. Self-medication via alcohol or even drugs can sometimes be a way to deal with stress, but we all know they are not a solution. Many tears have been shed in my office. A nutritionist's role is not only to guide the client towards his or her food choices and weight goals via coaching, but also to inspire and help him/her to get care of the "mind side" of the transformational journey.

I saw so many women coming to my group classes crying of exhaustion, desperate for a change, paralyzed by fear also at the prospect of changing. These women were often overwhelmed with stress. They arrived at the class completely frazzled, or they had missed the previous session because, as usual, there was something more important than themselves. I lost a few women in my group this way, because work or family was always coming first and they could not commit to a once a week evening meeting with us, or I should say themselves.

Picture yourself one day this week. How was your stress level? Very high or relatively low? Have you never lived days or moments where you were running like a chicken without a head, going from one task to another without stopping for one minute? You become dissociated from your body and feelings, and this can lead to depression and worse. You have no attention span left because you are already worrying about the next thing you need to do or a future event that has not even happened yet. What I have noticed with my groups is that when you ask participants to observe their stress level during one week sometimes they come back and say that had not really realized how stressed they were!

With this level of constant stress, you have this feeling that this is not the life you dreamt of, that in fact there is "a life" taking place outside of yourself, not YOUR life. When I had my first signs of burn-out, I remember having out-of-body moments. I was leaving my body and dissociating with myself. I was literally looking at myself, puzzled and lost. The doctor told me my mind was trying to escape my reality. I just wanted to flee, but I was paralyzed. Stress was eating me alive.

How many more chores or activities can you sandwich in a day, how many more hours can your employer demand?

Think about it. It is not just work. We have complicated our lives so much too. My mother never went to the hairdresser, or maybe once in a while to cut her hair. No bleaching, highlighting, or coloring. She did not have pedicures and manicures. She did not go to the gym or have a trainer, she did not go shopping often. Her clothes closet was very small, only a few dresses and suits. She had only one travel suitcase. We had one car and one TV. I can continue like this for another chapter about all the "stuff" we did not have or the things we did not do. And we had money. Yet we were content, happy and free most of the time. And by the way we were also skinny.

We have reached a point in our civilization where we have accumulated so much and have added so many activities in our lives that we are being suffocated. The working days get longer, so how much can you cram in the remaining hours? And if you do not have a job outside the home, is your life really that easier? Of course it is not. This nonstop race creates unhappiness, a feeling of void that is often filled with food. The reality is that our lives now are a collection of stressful events sprinkled with short moments of rest or pleasure. There is no such thing as a balanced life anymore.

However, there is a moment when you know you have reached your highest tolerance level. You must decide either to stay there and slide into more stress or to make a change. You may have finally crashed, and now have no other option than to change. This chapter is a wakeup call and an inspiration to take care of yourselves, my friends.

It is a cliché, but it is still very true. Women always put everybody ahead of themselves. The hubby comes back from work, exhausted, and announces he will go to a golf game with his friends. You on the other had plans to take a break with your girlfriends but grudgingly stay home for the kids. Again, this is not always true and there is balance and fluidity in gender roles now. Relationships can be fair. But my clients are mostly in their 50's to 70's and maybe, like me, belong to another generation where it was still true. Let me be honest. I have helped so many women now. I have encountered very few who could say they had a balanced life. It felt for most of them, even these in their 40's that they had to juggle the mom, the wife, the career and the care taker roles all at once. So, repeat after me:

Cogni-Tip:

There will be always someone or something bulldozing your agenda.

The reality of stress is that it is bad for everything: your health, your professional success, your relationships and spirituality. The first step is to realize where you are on the stress barometer:

Stress Level Barameter

LEVELS OF STRESS		
Level 1: Feels great, bliss, calm, happiness	↑	
Level 2: Feels good	*This is where you want to be*	
Level 3: Feels a little stressed but not bad stress	↓	
Level 4: Feels stressed, difficult to focus, worried		
Level 5: Overwhelmed, very stressed, irrational, wants to flee		

If you are in Level 1 or 2, you are doing pretty well. In fact, Level 1 is almost nirvana, and as the saying goes, you can never stay there too long because then you do not feel happiness anymore. You need to be stressed out and unhappy from time to time to appreciate these moments of bliss. I have to say it takes a lot of self-awareness work to totally realize these moments of happiness. Unfortunately, I believe that constant Facebooking and texting takes these moments away. Why go to a museum to take pictures of paintings? Why don't you just stop and really look at the beauty of the colors, the symbolism hidden in the painting and the mystery behind the subject? Just stop and smell the roses. Truly, I have learned to do that.

As I was writing this chapter in Boston, I took a stroll through Harvard Square and almost fell down. A young lady was taking pictures of the buildings as she was walking and she hit me. She did not stop to admire the buildings. She just took pictures. Was she really in the moment? She looked as if the pictures were more important than anything else. There are moments in my life, sometimes for months in a row that I now realize were the happiest times in my life. I vividly remember a Thanksgiving at home. When I went to bed after the party I felt a surge of profound happiness and gratitude for this moment we shared with friends and family. I was in the moment.

Level 3: Now, when you get to Level 3, you feel the stress, but not nonstop. You have the usual, even positive, stress related to a deadline to meet, a project you need to accomplish, a charged day or a flight to take (how stressful these days!). Maybe a little too much to do at once with conflicting priorities. But the next day everything goes back to normal. This is the flow of life with its mountains and valleys.

The danger starts at Level 4. This is where I was my friends, for too long. Repeat after me:

Cogni-Tip:

You cannot stay in Level 4 for too long! You need to learn to de-stress!

Level 4 is pretty intense. It is nonstop. You start to lose your focus. It is Level 3 without a break. You have an ever-growing to-do list that adds to your anxiety because you never see the end of it. Your schedule is cranked up to maximum level. You need to schedule your conversation with your mother at 4 p.m. every Friday, otherwise the window of opportunity is missed, how sad. You run from one kid's activity to the other. You arrive disheveled and late at your yoga session and are so stressed you do not even benefit from it. You run after the yoga session to pick the kids again and go buy a roasted chicken because there is no time to cook at home. You need to help your kids with their homework and prepare your business trip for tomorrow. Your partner is not available for babysitting, so you need to find somebody to take care of the kids the next day. But the usual person is sick, so you need to devise a plan C. You arrive at your business meeting unprepared because you did not sleep that well for the past two days. I can go on and on and on about a day like this…

Getting back to resilience. Some of you will do better for longer. Some of you will crash earlier. Some of you will develop ulcers, heart palpitations, anxiety disorders, or you may start to self-medicate with cookies, drinks, or worse. You can decide to slow down, change jobs, take a break - if you can – go to the gym and start running (this is what I did). But if you don't, you will go to **Level 5, or hell as I call it.**

Stress at Level 5 is the bottom, the end of the journey. You want to fight, or flee. BUT YOU CAN'T.

I remember thinking, when I was at Level 5, but not even yet able to realize it, that I wanted to die or disappear. I thought about fleeing the family coop. One night, after one of my girls asked me something about a new activity she wanted to start, I just flew the house, went into the woods next door and shouted a primal scream. And then I cried and sobbed and fell on the forest floor, under a tree. This was before the big breakdown. It was coming. I wanted to flee my life! In this stage you are becoming unable to really connect with others, you lose your focus, your become irrational, sloppy in your work. You do not have any energy left to love, especially yourself. You cannot stay at Level 5. It is destruction stage.

At Level 4 and 5, you experience what our bodies have been engineered to do for thousands of years: survive or die. If you stay petrified in front of a ferocious beast you will be devoured. It is fight of flight.

It was the encounter with the tiger or the fight with the enemy—when we lived in caves—that triggered these reactions. We did not live that stressfully, at least not every minute, in the not so distant past. But the survival skills we were gifted with by nature required strong actions. When in a fight of flight situation the whole body is triggered by certain hormones to deliver extra nutrients to the legs and arms muscles that are supposed to be used to run or combat. The senses are heightened, the heart is beating faster to pump blood to the heart, and to feed the muscles.

Flight or fight situations trigger hormones such as adrenaline and cortisol. Glucose, proteins, fats in your body are mobilized to deliver energy to the muscles, including the brain. Heart rate, breathing, blood circulation, body temperature increase to deliver oxygen and nutrients to muscles with a priority to arms and legs. The digestive system shuts down (not a priority when you are struggling). All the senses are heightened to help you SURVIVE.

However, in today's current lifestyle, we fight or flee all the time. It's not with a beast—

unless this is what your boss or partner is to you—it is with the traffic, the commute, the job, the deadlines, the kids, the partner, the family issues, the financial burden, the queue at the cash register—too slow, the verbal aggressions which are more and more frequent, the political divide and the anxiety about the future.

Unbeknownst to you, this never-ending stress situation affects all parts of your body:

- Your immune system is weakened hence the cold after a stressful event. And for some cancer may show up after a major stressful event in your life.
- Your energy level goes down
- Your sex drive takes a dive
- Your brain power is affected. Concentration, memory and focus are diminished. Errors become more frequent. You can become disengaged.

In a nutshell, stress gets internalized, if not evacuated, by affecting almost all your organs. Stress is responsible most of diseases, or at least it accelerates the process. It accelerates aging tremendously. Look at our U.S. Presidents after only four years in the White House. How terribly aged they look. Stress affects your brain by killing neurons at an accelerated pace. It triggers ulcers, insomnia, heart attacks, mental diseases and cancer. Stress is a life's robber in all ways possible, from the mental, to the physical and the emotional points of view.

Besides, and Here it Comes, Stress Makes You Fat Three Ways!

#1 Reason - Blame it on Cortisol:

Why, you say? It is due to a very complex cascade of hormones release. To keep it simple cortisol, a stress hormone, will help summon all possible stored glucose in your body in your blood for delivery of all your cells.

But the glucose is not used! Remember, you are nor running nor fighting! It has to be stored again! And what happens, insulin is released to transport it back to your storage, and once filled, as glycogen mostly in muscles and the liver, the rest is stored AS FAT!

So each time you get stress, you store fat. Even if you pay attention to what you eat, you gain weight inexplicably!

In the adipose tissues (where we store body fat) fatty acids are released in response to corti-sol.Long term exposure to too much cortisol reduces cellular sensitivity to insulin, a condition that is called "Syndrome X" or "Metabolic Syndrome" and is a precursor to diabetes. Because the role of cortisol is to encourage the body to refuel itself after a stress occurrence, our appetite increases (with a predilection for carbohydrates).

Leptin is another hormone that regulates our appetite. It tells you to stop eating when you are satiated. The reason I only believe in slow weight loss is because if you lose too much weight quickly, as in some shows on TV, your body goes into defense mode. Your body does not like to lose all this weight. It wants to replenish its treasure chest of fat. To do so, it lowers your leptin level, which makes you eat more because you feel satiated much later than usual.

#2 Reason – Your Brain Wants to Be Happy!

The brain wants to be happy. The brain does not like stress, unhappiness, trauma or grief. The brain will try to find happiness many different ways. This is why some of us take anti-depres-sants. They help remediate for the lack of serotonin, our happy feeling neurotransmitter. Dopa-mine, another neuro-transmitter also has a role in making us happy. It is a very complicated ballet in your brain.

When we are unhappy we may turn to food, especially sugar, for relief because it helps trigger extra neurotransmitters in your brain. A tough time at home today and a fight with a friend? Let's have a pastry with hot chocolate. There will be pleasure derived from this experience, unfor-tunately short lived, hence the potential never ending cravings - remember the chapter on sugar. Sugar calls for more sugar. After the pastry and the chocolate, there could be a few pretzels, fol-lowed by an ice cream.

A study led by Connecticut College students and a professor of psychology have found "America's favorite cookie" is just as addictive as cocaine for rats. Joseph Schroeder, associate professor of psychology and director of the behavioral neuroscience program, and his students found that"rats formed an equally strong association between the pleasurable effects of eating Oreos and a specific environment as they did between cocaine or morphine and a specific environ-ment. They also found that eating cookies activated more neurons in the brain's "pleasure center" than exposure to drugs of abuse."[1]

1: https://www.conncoll.edu/news/news-archive/2013/student-faculty-research-suggests-oreos-can-be-compared-to-drugs-of-abuse-in-lab-rats.html#.WcVcE7pFxZU

#3 Reason – Your Survival Mode is Hijacking Your Logical Brain

Remember the Fight of Flight situation. When you are in this situation, all logic goes through the roof. Your survival instincts, coming from what we call your older brain, or reptilian brain, is taking over. Do not, I repeat, do not go in a pastry shop during one of these moments.

Willpower, all the CogniDiet® positive thoughts, the healthy resolutions go haywire. There will be damage. You are not going to go to a salad bar. You will go for the sugar, as explained earlier because your body wants glucose to fight a non-existing fight. Your logical brain usually loses that battle. This is why willpower is not enough to change eating habits. You can resist it only for so long. It is a long and methodical process of deep change that will help you rewire your brain and adopt new behaviors that YOU MUST LOVE in order to stick with them.

Now You Know Why You Need to Address Stress!

On the stress scale we oscillate between these levels all the time. It is crucial however to never stay at Level 4 or 5 for too long. I read many books about stress reduction and methods to keep you grounded and sane. I myself had to undergo therapy in 2006 to get out of my burnout and associated depression. My therapist used CBT and advised me to start meditation. I started to research ways to calm myself down, besides the fact I was taking an antidepressant. I discovered running and hired a meditation coach. This was my way of coping with my stress.

If you are feeling over-stressed, don't despair, there are many ways we can address it and cope with it. There are drastic solutions, but there are also tips and short-term fixes that I myself still use from time to time when the stress level is getting to 4 for too long.

Let's start with of course the radical life changing solutions. And let's face it, deep down, some of you know that some big issues, which are huge stressors, need to be addressed. It could be:

- I need a new career. I must quit this crazy job!
- I must leave this toxic partner
- I need to get my financial status in order
- I must face my demons, whatever they are and seek therapy

However, these are all easier said than done. I have witnessed career changes, divorces, initiation of psycho-therapy and going back to school decisions, which are major milestones in a life. Some of my clients were ready for the big change. But everybody is at a different stage when contemplating change. It requires courage to start afresh. The weight loss is usually a first step in the transformative process.

Let's explore some short-term options to deal with stress. There are the practical solutions such as baby steps in changing jobs. You are for instance selecting one with a shorter commute. Or the decision to stop volunteering for so many committees and task forces.

INSTANT Cogni-Shift:

One of the easiest ways to lower your stress level is to learn to say **NO!** Do it a few times this week.

Write a list of all the things you could eliminate right now from your life:

_____

_____

_____

_____

_____

Now calculate how much time this elimination list will give back to you, to:
- Exercise
- Walk
- Have a weekly massage
- Meditate
- Attend a weight loss support group
- Take a new class online to further my education etc.

I now have _____ hours back into my week to take care of ME! And darn it, I deserve it!

Cogni-Game:

Make a bold resolution right now, in this moment. What will you do this week for yourself? Write it down immediately and make it visible to you.

I will

_____

By now in this chapter I want you to start thinking about potential life changes, and/or baby steps to lower your stress level. However, it is not that easy, for some of you, to even begin to change.

My hope for you is that at least you realize at what level of stress you are. Being able to identify what state you are in is the first step to come up with tools to manage it. There are small techniques that can help you calm your brain - remember that we oscillate between these different stress levels.

You cannot decide to leave a meeting that is contentious and go running. You cannot yell at somebody because you feel frustrated. You cannot quit your job on a whim. You want to stay calm and think about your options. Building awareness about your situation, sources of stress and potential solutions is what you must focus on. It will allow you to move from a world of emotions to a world of action. Besides, you bought this book because you want to lose weight!

Cogni-Tip:

Remember stress will trigger sugar cravings!

There are different ways to calm yourself down. Remember the first thing is to realize at what level you are.

Describe at what level you were between Level 1 and 5. Or look at a few different days in the week and assess your overall situation.

Moment in the Day	Stress Level	Why?
Example: At 4 p.m. my daughter came back from abroad. I picked her up at the airport. I had not seen her for 4 months.	Level 1, I am in heaven. But just before that I was at Level 3, just a little bit stressed about finding a parking spot at the airport.	Pure happiness Fear of being late when she arrives
Example: Monday at 3 p.m., I was in a contentious meeting. I did not agree with my boss but had to support him/her.	Level 4. This difficult situation has lasted the whole week.	I am not myself. This is very uncomfortable as I feel I have to lie to cover him/her.
Use this template to write your own situations and stress levels.		

If you discover that you are in level 3 to 5 for 80% of the time, you know you need to do something about it. If you are this girl, and you are packing pounds, you may also think about addressing the issue seriously as YOU KNOW it is impacting your health as well. I recommend that you start meditating. It saved my sanity and I am absolutely certain it saved my brain. Meditation rewired my brain and created new happiness pathways. My personality has been completely transformed since I crashed and took care of myself. I am a happier, more positive, and more self-aware person.

In the meantime, it is imperative to help you calm down, on the spot, immediately. There are different methods that I teach and encourage in my class:

1. The visualization method
2. The trick your brain method
3. The learn to breathe method

Method #1: The Visualization Method

I discovered Dr. Laurel Mellin's book "Wired for Joy" and her technique for Emotional Brain Training or EBT a few years ago. Her premise is that we must make our brain happy. Here is a link to her EBT website: www.ebtconnect.net.   Her principles are that if you can give a happy moment to your brain, it will calm down. It is like watching a horror movie but in reverse. In fact, she says, we can fool our brain. If you watch a scary movie, you know it's not real, yet your fight of flight reflexes are triggered. You shout, your close your eyes, your heartbeat increases, your palms are sweating. You may even flee the movie theater. The truth is that your brain is not as smart as it looks. Your brain could not really see the difference between fiction and reality. So if you can picture or imagine a feel happy movie, your brain will feel happy instead of scared. Clifford Lazarus, Ph.D., as we worked together on this book told me that "the mind and body are two different sides of the same coin and they intersect most profoundly at the level of imagination." We can powerfully influence almost all of the physical systems of the body by using specific visualization techniques.

She recommends summoning a picture that reminds you of a very happy moment. It must be extremely vivid. You need to leverage all your senses to imagine:

- The smells
- The way the person is dressed, the colors and patterns of the clothes, the texture of the hair
- Or, if you don't summon a person(s), what is the moment about, the location, the scenery etc.
- Is there noise around you? Is it on a beach, in a meadow?
- You need to think about everything like if you were back in that moment

Dr. Mellin says that it usually involves a mother-child bond as it is the strongest feeling of love. Most of my clients will summon a picture of their child(ren) or parents. It can also be a moment where you feel you transcended yourself, like when you climbed your first mountain, or built a house for Habitat for Humanity, volunteered in Africa to teach children etc.

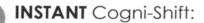

INSTANT Cogni-Shift:

So what is your moment of extreme happiness?

My moment of extreme happiness is:

_____

This is mine. The day my two girls, Camille and Pauline, rejoined me after three months of separation when we moved to the United States from Belgium. At that time, in 1995, you could still get to the gates and welcome family and friends. I remember them jumping in my arms right out of the gate. I remember the way they were dressed. They were each holding a huge stuffed dalmatian their aunt had given them before departure. They ran to me shouting "Mama!" What a wonderful moment. It was not only the reunion. It was the fact we were starting a new chapter in our life, a life in a new country, with a new job. With a new job that would allow me to spend more time with them - and it did initially for 3 wonderful years in Atlanta. A life that was more relaxed and where we had dinners together. I had time to go to their school plays, and we had wonderful weekends. The kids also have fantastic memories of this time in our lives.

Method #2: "Trick your brain" to think about something else.

In this case, you try to calm your brain by focusing on something else. You engage your brain in an exercise of observation. Look at the room around you, or the environment, and decide to focus on an object. It can be a vase of flowers, a tree, a car or a clock on the wall. This method is very useful when you really cannot leave a situation, and cannot even close your eyes to visualize your favorite moment or do a mini meditation. I use this method a lot when I was trapped in a meeting and was feeling a panic attack coming. In a less dramatic situation, if you feel a craving for sugar is coming, distract yourself with something. You will see that usually the craving will go away after a few minutes, because you re-directed your brain into another direction.

Now describe this object to yourself. Think about all the elements that compose an object. You can go very technical or poetic on this one!

- The shape
- The colors, textures, fabric or materials etc.
- How does it work, when was it made, who may have made it etc.

By doing this exercise, you deflect your brain's attention from stress—which is emotional and usually irrational—to a logical and methodical experiment that will calm the emotional side of the moment. You replace emotion with rationalism if you will. Of course, if you are in a car accident or another major stressful event, you will not be thinking about this. However do not underestimate the power of calming your brain.

Method #3: Learn to Breathe

Most of the time, when you are stressed, you forget to breathe correctly. You usually only engage the upper side of your lungs. You breathe shallowly. The consequences are that you do not supply enough oxygen to your brain. Lack of oxygen does not help with calming down or trying to stay in control and logical.

There are also other benefits to breathing correctly. Breathing correctly activates the hypothalamus, which is connected to the pituitary gland in the brain. It sends out hormones that inhibit stress-producing substances such as adrenaline for instance. Breathing also triggers a relaxation response in the body and enhances Alpha waves creation in the brain. Alpha brain are proven to promote pain relief, lower stress and promote wellbeing. Alpha waves are produced when in a state of semi wakefulness or in a meditative state. This is one of the reasons meditation is recommended to people with high stress levels. Finally breathing brings extra oxygen to the brain obviously and redirects attention to your body versus the event or environment around you.

Here are a couple of techniques. Just slowing down and breathing mindfully is enough to calm you down. The beauty of this exercise is that you can do it anywhere, any moment. You can perform it discreetly and nobody will notice.

Technique #1: Count to 4

- Breathe through your nose and put your hands on your belly
- Feel your lungs entirely when inhaling– not just the upper part, and count to 4
- Hold your breath, count to 4
- Exhale slowly and count to 4 as you exhale
- Feel your belly rising and dropping while you do the exercise
- Repeat this cycle 4 times

Technique #2: The alternative nostril breathing

It is the same but you close one nostril and inhale with the other. Then you exhale with the other one. This forces you to inhale more forcefully. And the alternation deflects your attention from stress to the mechanical aspect of breathing.

There are other techniques to relax!

I recommend the body scan. Again, it helps you to get re-grounded in your own body. You close your eyes, and scan each section of your body for tension and relax. It is recommended to start with the toes. Let go of the tension you may feel in that part of your body at that moment. You can be as granular as you want with each body part, ending with the crown of your head. It can be a quick 10-minute total body scan or you can make it last longer. Start the experiment in your bedroom or in a very comfortable chair.

Mini meditation sessions are also beneficial and can be associated with breathing, without the need to go to any class to learn how to meditate. You rhythm your breathing and associate each phase with words that are being whispered when you inhale and exhale. For instance you can use the word "peace" on the inhale and "let go" on the exhale. This requires more privacy of course but helps you retain good energy and let go of negative feelings.

And then of course there is the "distraction list" that allows your body and mind to focus on something else, like engaging in a conversation, taking a walk, playing music or drawing. Write yours and practice it.

In the resource section of this book, you will find some useful apps that I recommend for meditation or self- relaxation.

Cogni-Tip:

Make it a habit to relax regularly, even for a few minutes, during the day. Your brain and health need it.

You will be surprised at how much more productive you will be and how much your stress level may abate. However if you have a tough life and your stress is unbearable I want you to learn from me. Don't crash. You will need to address it sooner or later. In this chapter I will share my own story about dealing with stress and learning to conquer it.

There are no experiments this week!

I want no added distractions. I just want you to apply what I have been sharing in this chapter. Take a break, have a massage, go for a long walk and reflect on your life. Note your stress level at different moments of the days and make a few decisions regarding what needs to be weeded out. Don't forget to think about toxic relationships, energy vampires, and unnecessary activities and think hard about your happiness factor as you make your decisions.

Write your plan, short and longer term, to eliminate stress:

_____

_____

_____

_____

Now, My Story

I am not here to lecture anybody on how they should lead their life. Life is complicated. Our society has made it more stressful every year. But there is always help; let's be optimistic. If you are more fragile than others, my best advice besides potential pharmacological help (believe me an anti-depressant can make a big difference) is to join a support group. Being able to speak openly and freely, and getting non-judgmental advice and help can make a huge difference because you feel you are not alone anymore in your struggle. If you look for help, it will come. Don't despair.

I believe having spent 11 years in boarding school from a very young age gave me the pugnacity and grits of a fighter because every day was a battle for the best seat at the cafeteria, or to be with the right "gang" in the dorm rooms etc. In its own way, you can be fragile and tough at the same time. So after a few minutes of self-pitying sometimes, I usually rebound, slap myself and stop complaining. I am a lucky girl, I have been blessed with many gifts in my life. One is resilience, definitely.

The decision to start The CogniDiet® was my way to give back to other women and help them transform. Because make no mistake, this program is not just about weight loss. The weight loss is the physical proof of the transformation. I am a big women's power advocate kind of girl. I am for women putting themselves first. Cause we deserve it, darn it! At The CogniDiet®, we witnessed new careers blossoming, new boyfriends or girlfriends appearing, renewed optimism and hope in our participants' spirit. This program, as I see it, is a great "support group" for women who want to change. The weight loss is a metaphor for pruning your life. It is the excess baggage that goes when we let life in and go with the flow of our vital forces.

It is only when I had the courage to face my limitations, which was very hard, that I knew at the ripe age of 52 that I had to change my life. I had to go to Level 5 to crash and burn to finally resurrect from my ashes. I remember presenting a marketing plan to the highest level of management in my company and having a panic attack at that moment. I had to stop for a few seconds and re-collect my thoughts. I said: "can I start all over again". I cannot believe I did this. And I got away with it.

But my attention span and ability to focus were suffering. I knew my performance level was rapidly going down. I could sometimes catch the annoyed or worried look of one of my managers when I could not find a word. I blanked and looked lost. I suddenly left meetings to go and hide in the bathroom. I had panic attacks hitting me uncontrollably more frequently, haphazardly and greater in intensity. A panic attack is like a fake heart attack and for me it always started with tingling in my toes and then a wave of adrenaline was going through my body. The brain at that moment shuts down.

I started to withdraw, even from family, and kept everything bottled up and secret. The panic attacks became so frequent that I had to take a leave of absence. I saw the family doctor who sent me to a fantastic psychiatrist and a psychologist. The psychiatrist told me I was at the very bottom of self-destruction. A couple of more weeks and I would have been hospitalized. I could also have killed myself.

I never felt so much like a failure, a miserable bundle of weakness. I believe my ego had been totally shattered. As I said, at the bottom, there are only two ways out. I decided to take care of myself.

Besides therapy and medication, I started to meditate and run. I ended up running at least 5 times a week. I lost a lot of weight and looked very fit as my brain was healing. It's funny, but when you are "sick" like this in your head and look very good, people are very puzzled. You look your healthiest while being miserable inside. This is why you can fool people for so long.

The running became a meditative activity. I always went along the canal and basked into the beauty of the water, the rays of sun between the leaves, the trees and the many animals I encountered. In Japan it's called a "forest bath."

I Faced My Limitations and Took Action

I re-assessed my skills and abilities and faced the truth. I was not cut for the high-level career in the big corporation anymore. I had reached my mental incompetence level aha! There was something too soft about me. I was not cut for the cynical decisions, the cut-throat battles, the coldness of numbers and the limitations of a life mostly focused on the corporate rat race. This was my moment of truth. I had reached my maximum stress tolerance threshold. I knew it, and initially despised this realization.

I had to accept and deal with this softness. Becoming a nutritionist not only allowed me to take care of myself and change my life but also made me a better person. It allowed me to accept this softer and more compassionate side of me that thrives on helping people. ALL PEOPLE. Not just the high performers, the bosses and the critical colleagues. All the women and men who need help with their health and weight. All the people who struggle with life as it is and need someone to listen to them, to guide them without judgement. People who can speak freely in a group or in the sanctuary of my office without the risk of being labeled, classified, judged or discarded like in a professional performance review.

My life is risky; I have to work hard, but I love it. And I lost the weight by taking care of myself, mostly for my brain's health initially. My heart has blossomed and I let out all the good things I have to offer. It does not mean that I live in la-la land either. I have a business to run, a bottom line to achieve. I have a vision for my program and ambition to help many, many people. But

I have merged my spiritual purpose and my life responsibilities. I am still driven and ambitious, I want to make money, I want to succeed but I do it at a different pace. My pace.

Be inspired my friends. Think about all the talents and gifts that have been bestowed upon you. Dig deep and find out how you can align your desired heart-centered purpose and your life responsibilities. Deal with your stress and brush your teeth every day.

And yes, I do what I preach. I do the breathing, I meditate and I exercise. I say no to too many parties or activities. I stop working and take a break when I know I need it. I monitor my stress level. I stopped building never ending to-do lists. I will never let myself go in Level 5 again. I have not taken an anti-depressant for almost 7 years now. But I would take it again if I needed to. I finally know who I am.

CogniDiet® Book Club Discussion Guide

This week was about stress relief. I hope your week was OK CogniGirls®! I also hope that you have made a priority to attend these meetings with your partners in crime. Friendship, group support and working together towards the same goals is essential for your mental balance. In fact this is why I started the CogniDiet® group setting and used it for my clinical trial. These women were all very busy women but took the time to meet once a week for twelve weeks. If they could do it, you can too.

- **Where is your stress level at most of the time?**

- **Is this a typical week for you in terms of stress level?**

- **Have you done something for yourself this week to relax or just wind down?**

- **Have you used the visualization or breathing techniques?**

- **What have you decided to do to about your stress level? For the short term, and the long term?**

- **Have you eliminated some activities?**

- **How are you doing in general with your weight loss goals? Better than you thought or do you need more support from the group? How can they help you?**

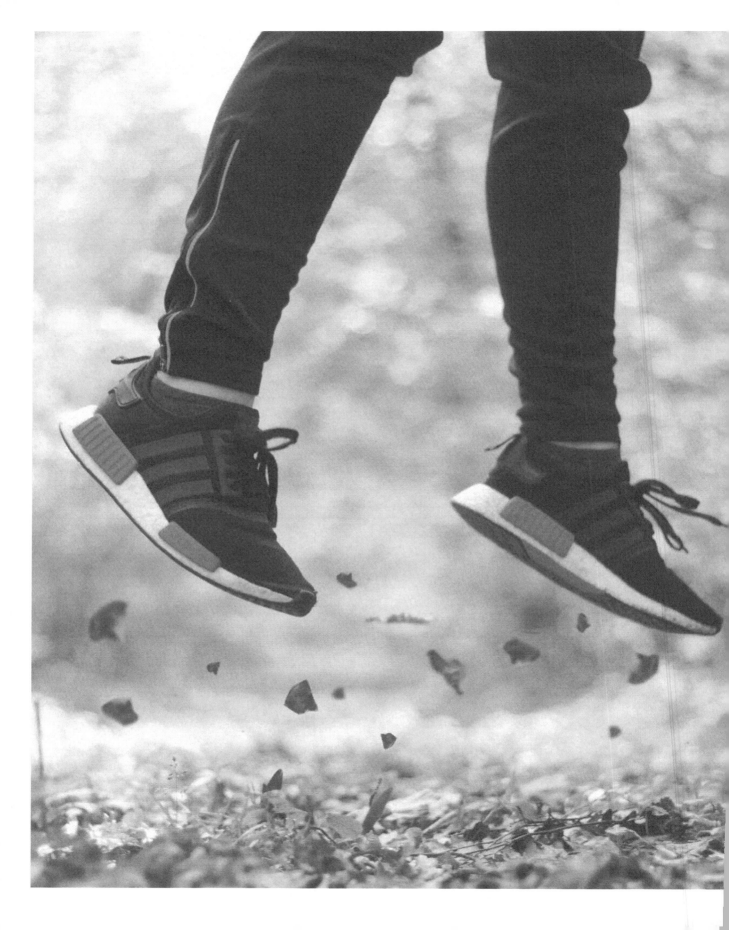

Chapter 6

I Am a Mean, Fat-Burning Machine!

Muscles Are the New Sexy!

You are going to say, "Finally, she covers exercise!" Remember: 80% of weight loss is due to nutrition and food choices. We cover exercise at a later stage in the 12-week curriculum because I want participants to first think about changing their eating behaviors without relying on exercise to counteract a potentially excessive food intake. Susan, a fitness trainer and friend of mine, shared her wisdom pearl with us on day:

"You Can Never Outrun Your Fork!"
- Fitness Trainer Susan Panzica, Princeton

Cogni-Tip:

The sweating and building of muscles will absolutely help with weight loss—and overall health—as we are burning calories, but the discipline with food choices must come first.

Now, let's examine exercise as an activity: do you love it or hate it; do you feel neutral about it or do you fear it? Do you exercise consistently or not at all? Do you mix cardiovascular and strength training? Do you know what HIIT or MHR mean? Is it easy for you to get moving or are you a couch potato? Are you genetically gifted with muscles—yes there is a gene for that!

FEAR NOT MY FRIEND! I will, I'm sure, convince you exercise is a worthwhile investment of your precious time. And more importantly, it is NEVER too late to start exercising. You will be motivated by the story of Daphne, an incredibly fit and muscular 75-year-old woman who lost 23 pounds with me in three years and has gone from a 35% to a 25% body fat ratio! In my clinical trial women were not very high on the exercise activity level, to start with. When I met them for the six-month follow-up, they had to fill in a questionnaire. They indicated an average increase from almost none to 3 days of exercise a week. And I witnessed this transformation looking at their body shape, not just their weight shift. Now some of you I know, will say "I hate exercise, I will never like it, don't lecture me. I do it just because I have to." Maybe I can help you enjoy it a little bit more?

What Are Your Excuses?

When I came in the U.S. in 1995, I was still pretty skinny, but found multiple reasons not to exercise. I'm not the only one who finds reasons to avoid it; here are a few excuses I've collected from clients over the years, some of them pretty funny. Maybe you will recognize yours:

- I am too tired—definitely the #1 excuse
- I just have 30 minutes, not enough to go to the gym
- I have a meeting tonight
- I am busy with the kids. I want to be with my kids, I don't see them enough
- We have a party/meeting, I need to look good and I can't be sweaty
- I can't exercise, I just went to the hairdresser
- I want to lose weight before I dare showing my body at the gym (yeah right!)
- I have to stay late at the office/church/school /fill in the blank
- I just ate
- I did not shave my legs
- I have an unexpected appointment (really?)
- I don't look good in my gym attire, yet (yes, this one!)
- It's too late, it's too early, it's too hot, it's too cold, it's raining, it's snowing
- It's a Holiday
- I have visitors
- I am traveling etc.

Chronic fatigue was, in retrospect, my number one excuse. When I began training seriously I was literally crawling to the gym in the evening. I did not want to go. I found, especially in the winter, that if I went directly from the train station to home I could not leave again. I collapsed on the couch and cuddled with my kids. I enjoyed my home's familiar cocooning surroundings after battling the subway and train. Snuggling into the sofa was like going back in my mother's womb. But then, I learned to keep my gym attire in the car and go directly from the train station to the club. I also focused on how well I would feel after the session. Besides, after a few months, I saw such a body and energy transformation that it kept me motivated.

I stuck to my intention because I penned it in my calendar and took it as seriously as a business meeting or a doctor's appointment. And, instead of "Exercise or gym," I wrote "Feel good session" in my agenda. I mentally experienced, through visualization, what I was getting out of it: a muscular body, stronger legs, more defined arms, less stress, happy endorphins in my brain, loving myself and being proud of my transformation. Even if you are a couch potato, just start by walking and increase the time and the difficulty (think gentle hills) week after week. Or enroll in a beginner's yoga class. Look at this new activity from a stress relief point of view.

INSTANT Cogni-Shift:

> Find something you like to do, please try, and look at it from a stress relief point of view. This will change the way you look at exercise. Don't use the word "exercise." Just use the word "fun activity."

So Many Good Things Happen When You Are on the Move!

How can we inspire you to start being more active and stop thinking about exercise as a chore? Maybe using other words to describe it would help such as activity, moving, or having fun? Or using CBT, you can motivate yourself by thinking about all the health and physical amazing benefits it brings to your life:

- Release of feel-good endorphins a.k.a. the runner's high
- Promotion of blood micro-circulation, important for your brain!
- Improvement of lymphatic drainage, important for general elimination
- Stress relief and to some people, a form of meditation
- Sweating the toxins out
- Burning glucose (all these carbs you eat) and fat
- Strengthening the heart muscle
- Oxygenating the whole body
- Building muscles
- Continuing to burn extra calories, even after exercising, up to 48 hours
- Proven to:
  - ✓ Increase longevity and quality of life by slowing cellular aging
  - ✓ Lower blood glucose and hemoglobin A1c
  - ✓ Lower cholesterol
  - ✓ Burn body fat
  - ✓ Lower blood pressure
  - ✓ Lower depression mood

INSTANT Cogni-Shift:

Think about how well you will feel — all these benefits — after a good hour of sweating or just moving (even walking outside). Close your eyes and visualize the benefits

How much exercise you begin with depends on the shape you are currently in. You either need to start exercising, or you need to boost your current regimen. Sometimes you can be stuck in a rut, even if you go to the gym three times a week. If you always do the same routine your body gets acclimated and does not burn as many calories anymore. Therefore, you will burn less calories. Or, if you have cut your food intake too drastically, and added intensive exercising all of a sudden, your body will feel starved and hold on to its fat reserves as a protection.

INSTANT Cogni-Shift:

What is your new slogan, benefit or motivational quote to boost your current exercise/activity regimen? Go back to your vision board. What was your inspiration there?

Write your motto starting with the word "I" and make this visible every day like a special vision board. These will be your new PATs:

Example:

Exercise to me: I love this feeling of greater mental clarity I get after I go running outside. I can solve problems so much easier after a good run. I feel so refreshed. I also feel more optimistic.

What is yours? And if you do not exercise at all, find a way to describe how you feel or could feel after one hour of your preferred activity, like just walking…

Now that you have done this, it is time to start looking at what exercise, or just being more active, can really do for you as far as weight loss is concerned.

How Much Do I Need to Burn to Lose a Pound?

Let's examine how exercise can help you burn fat. It takes an average of 3,500 calories to burn a pound of fat. One pound of fat a week. This calculation was questioned however by a paper published in The Lancet, by The National Institutes for Health (NIH), August 26, 2011. They believe we may, as we age and as our metabolism and muscle mass decline, need to burn as high as 7,000 calories.

But I believe this is a little bit extreme. My philosophy is to cut calories, with a reasonable yet long term view. We are talking about 500 – 700 calories a day. That is the ugly truth. Fat does not come off by just walking to the restroom once in a while being seated all day in front of your computer. And I say "average". For some of us it could be less or more pending our genetics, age, dieting history, muscle mass and current metabolism.

Are you going to run one hour to burn the extra muffin you just bought between dropping the kids at school and going to a meeting with your accountant? Are you going to swim an extra 45 minutes to eliminate the delicious Frappuccino you sipped in your car before you came home to cook dinner? No, you won't! It is much easier to acquire calories than burn them.

How can you reverse your mental pathways from the word "consuming" to "burning" calories and associate this new behavior with the word "pleasure?" How can you burn an extra 3,500 calories a week to start with, and then maintain a healthy weight?

What you can burn, as an average, for one hour of exercise/average for a 150 pound woman:

Energy You Use, Calories You Burn

Level	Type	Calories/Hour
Light activity 1 hour	• Lying down/ sleeping/sitting • House cleaning • Yoga (gentle)	• 60-100 • 180 • 200
Moderate activity 1 hour	• Gardening, walking, golfing, lawn mowing • Swimming (1/4 mile/hr) walking faster • Weight lifting, roller skating, soccer, hockey, etc.	• 220-250 • 250-300 • 300+
Vigorous activity 1 hour	• Ice skating, tennis (single), very fast walking, biking or running (15 min/mile) • Rowing machine, running (10 min/mile) • Stair climbing, running (6 min/mile)	• 400 • 600 • 900

Depends on physical condition, endurance, ability, level of effort and difficulty, age, weight, etc. These are just averages.

Find Something You Like to Do

Find an activity that you have always wanted to learn. That is the secret to burn calories while being happy. A client in her fifties start kayaking. She even bought a new car to carry her new canoe. Another enrolled in ballroom dancing to train for her son's wedding and lost many pounds enjoying herself with her husband while practicing.

If you are already active, find something that will take it up a notch. As a runner I finally enrolled and trained for a half marathon in 2012. If you are a walker, start walking with ski poles. You will build muscles in your arms and burn 20% more calories. Or just take the stairs instead of the escalator. Park your car further from the shops. Buy a Fitbit® or any other calorie and activity counter and walk more. All these little tips can help you burn more calories even without exercising. But don't turn these victories and extra steps into permission to allow yourself to eat more!

Fun Activities My Clients Discovered:

- Ballroom dancing – Hello tango!
- Kayaking or rowing
- Trekking mountains
- Plant and mushroom foraging in the forest
- Hiking National Parks
- Aqua aerobics – so gentle for your joints
- Spinning
- Hot yoga
- Snow shoeing
- Scuba diving etc.

Write your new favorite activity — one you would like to discover — here:

Within the next two weeks, I will search/start to

_____

Muscles Are Your Weight Loss Best Friends

Besides finding your favorite activity you can also start to adopt some special strategies to build this new body of yours. Many women favor cardiovascular activities over strength training, which means muscle building. The reasons are always the same:

- I don't like working with weights — I don't like it either, to tell you the truth.
- I don't want to build bulk — a sad excuse but I heard it often
- I only want to exercise outside
- Gyms and equipment are dirty! All these microbes...
- I can only do this with a trainer and I have no budget
- I have a frozen shoulder, a hip problem, weak knees etc.
- I will gain weight — yes, I heard this one too! It's true that muscles weigh more than fat, but they occupy less volume.

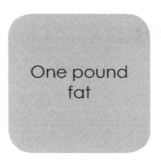

Cardiovascular activities are good for fat burning. They also help you strengthen your heart. Running a lot will build muscles in your legs. But in order to really build muscles, you need strength training. In spite of all the above excuses remember what a stronger body can do for you. In fact, when I combined strength training and running, I noticed I started to run faster.

Cogni-Tip:

What if I told you that more muscles will help you lose more weight? Isn't that an attractive proposition?

JUST BUILD MUSCLES, LADIES!
Why?

Because Muscle Mass Contributes 20% vs. 5% for Fat to Total Daily Energy Expenditure (TDEE)[1]

The more muscles you have the better your metabolism or ability to burn calories. However let's be realistic. Most of the TDEE or 80% is burned by your organs, 20% by your muscles and 5% by your fat (for people with a 20% body fat). So you would need to build 4 to 6 pounds of muscles over a period of a few months to be able to burn an extra 42 calories a day[1]. I am not going to say the more muscles, the more you can eat, but it is also true! Besides, after exercising,

1: Elia M. Organ and tissue contribution to metabolic rate. In: Kinney JM, Tucker HN (eds). Energy metabolism: tissue determinants and cellular corollaries. Raven: New York; 1992. pp 19–59.

muscles continue to burn calories up to 24 hours after exercising.

Ideally your body fat should be at 25%. Young people who are fit should be around 18-20%[2]. Don't push yourself too hard. Being at 32%[2] of body fat is officially classified as obese. What matters is to make it go down! Don't get discouraged if you start from this higher percentage. I try to get my clients to initially go under 30%.

Cogni-Tip:

Consider your muscles as an asset you have to protect. If you do not use them, you will lose them. If you work on them, they will grow again. It is never too late.

There are many ways we can lose muscle mass. You can witness it if you break a leg and wear a cast for a while. Your leg muscle mass is visibly melting. Astronauts who spend too much time in zero gravity come back very lean. They do not use their muscles, therefore they literally melt away. They have difficulty walking when they land back on earth. They have to be carried out of their landing pods and go for re-education. Besides being in space, there are many other more common reasons for losing muscle mass:

Reasons We Lose Muscles:

1. **Age:** we lose 0.5 to 1% of muscle mass every year after 50[3] if we don't do anything about it. The percentage of loss accelerates after you reach your forties.
2. **Lack of activity**, as said earlier
3. **Constant dieting**, without strength training! Triggers not only fat, but also muscles loss. A small study undertaken in Holland showed that fat-free mass accounted for 18% of weight loss in a very-low-calorie diet group and 7.7 % of weight loss in a low-calorie diet group, the study found.[4]

This will happen if you do not do proper strength exercise and eat enough protein while you are on a diet.

2: Jackson AS, Pollock ML., generalized equations for predicting body density of women. Med SC Sports Exerc. 1980;12(3):175-81

3: Phillips SM (July 2015). "Nutritional supplements in support of resistance exercise to counter age-related sarcopenia". Adv. Nutr. 6 (4): 452–460.

4: Roel Vink and Marleen van Baak, of the School for Nutrition, Toxicology and Metabolism at Maastricht University in the Netherlands, presented at the European Congress on Obesity in Bulgari, May 28, 2014.

Every time you undertake extreme dieting, your body will use its own reserves of fat and muscles for energy. This is one of the reasons constant dieters, who do not care about exercising, end up losing so much muscles mass that each time they go on a diet again their calorie burning machine is less effective. Genetics, exercise and diet history impact your mass of muscles, and even your ability to bulk them up. A study from 2000 published in the *Journal of Applied Physiology* found via body imaging testing, that women tend to have less muscle mass, closer to 30% of their body weight, while men have about 40%. This means an average woman of 150 pounds could have 45 pounds of muscles[5].

Cogni-Tip:

No. A pound of muscle does not burn 50 calories a day. It is a myth. One pound of muscles will burn an average of 4.5 to 7 calories a day vs. 4 times less for fat[1]. So if you can build an extra 6 pounds of muscles (replacing fat mass), you will burn an extra maximum of 42 calories per day. Not bad at all.

Being Smarter at Exercising

My last advice for this chapter is to exercise smarter. When I did the six-month follow up visits for my clinical trial in June 2016, I remember one participant particularly. When she began the program was exercising seven times a week, always following the same routine, mostly cardiovascular. She complained she was not losing weight anymore. She coupled this with cutting calories out of frustration. Guess what happened. She gained four pounds. She had forgotten the fact that the body adapts to monotonous exercising. It's like your brain. If you don't challenge yourself, there is no growth or change. She starved her body both ways.

Here is the magical "Open Sesame" key to unlock your frustrations and accelerate weight loss:

> High Intensity Interval Training or HIIT will get rid of your stubborn waist fat rolls!

5: Ian Janssen, Steven B. Heymsfield, ZiMian Wang, Robert Ross. Journal of Applied Physiology Published 1 July 2000 Vol. 89 no. 1, 81-88

I do HIIT with many clients to show how to do it the RIGHT WAY: 99% failed the test. HIIT principles are based on the fact that by boosting your heart for short periods of time you will put your body into a super fat burning machine mode. Oxygen and glycogen are not enough to fuel your heart rate. Fat is being burned. Most importantly, you create a form of extreme cellular stress, and your body has to recover so you will continue to burn more calories than usual for up to 24-48 hours.

During the intensive part of HIIT, you cannot talk, believe me. You cannot tell me you were busy selling a house a few minutes ago and had to run to the gym to meet me and by the way what could you eat tonight? You think you will die, you will explode. It has to stop very soon. And the good news is that it is intense, but very short. Multiple studies show that HIIT will help you lose more fat than any mild exercise activity[6].

Cogni-Tip:

I can make you a promise. Do this **two to three times a week** for 20 minutes and your fat will melt at a rate you've never seen it before. You can do this at any age, in any physical condition. You just have to learn to accelerate your heart rate to its maximum limit smartly and safely.

WARNING: Especially if you never exercised, or have health issues specifically with your heart, I do not want you to have a heart attack on the elliptical machine. Test yourself first, talk to your trainer and your physician. You need to know your limits.

HIIT training offers different modes and time cycles. It can be done on any machine or even while walking. You can research the internet to find its many different regimen. You have the 30 second burst and two minute cool off, or the one minute burst and three minute cool off, etc. You can also combine this with strength training. You will see results after one week!

My "aha" moment:
The less time I exercise, the quicker and the more weight I lose!

6: E.G.Trapp et al. The Effects of High Intensity Intermittent Exercise Training on Fat Loss and Fasting Insulin Levels of Young Women. International Journal of Obesity (2008) 32, 684-691.

Find Your Maximum Heart Rate

Before we embark on this you must find out your maximum heart rate, or MHR. There is a formula for this but MHR varies according to your genetics, physical condition, etc. For instance, mine at close to age 60 is 180 instead of 160. Why? Because I have exercised regularly for the past 13 years.

Here is the formula to help you:

> ## 220 – your age = your MHR
> As an example: 220 – 50 (age) = 170 beats per minute

You will see in the chart below that in order to be in the "losing weight" mode, which is called the anaerobic (lack of oxygen) and cardio fitness zones you must be at minimum 65% of your MHR.

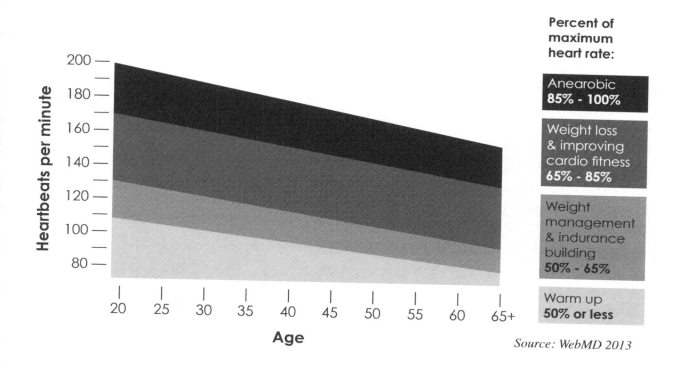

Percent of maximum heart rate:

Anearobic
85% - 100%

Weight loss & improving cardio fitness
65% - 85%

Weight management & indurance building
50% - 65%

Warm up
50% or less

Source: WebMD 2013

Let's calculate your zones – and calculate your MHR first

Zones	Your Numbers	Breathing and talking
Warm up	Less than 50% X MHR =	Normal and easy
Weight Management & Endurance	65% X MHR = 50% X MHR =	Challenging to talk and heavy breathing
Weight Loss & Improving Cardio Fitness	85% X MHR = 65% X MHR =	Conversation is extremely difficult
Anaerobic	100% X MHR = 85% X MHR =	You just can't talk anymore. This is also why this part of a HIIT is very short.

I highly recommend all of my clients, especially in their fifties or above, to carry a heart monitoring device. Many wearable devices now also include heart monitors. At the gym, when I don't feel like checking my watch all the time, I rely on the machine. I initially test the machine's heart monitoring system to find out if it's mimicking my own heartbeat. If I see it's rather reliable, I forget about my own device.

Once you get accustomed to doing HIIT, you will become extremely attuned to your heartbeat rhythm. You will be able to exercise intuitively by following your breathing pattern. I am red in the face like a tomato, disheveled, curly haired and sweaty after 30 minutes.

You can see from the above charts, that if you are "cruising" while exercising, you are not going to get into the super calorie burning mode offered by HIIT. Believe me, this boosted my weight loss results. It allowed me also to go to the gym for shorter periods.

I hope I have convinced you of the importance of building muscles and burning calories smartly. And no excuses, you can also do it while walking. You can do it at 80 years old, too.

Now, let's explore ways to get motivated to exercise, besides all the benefits we just covered. Again, the experiments I will share with you are the ways we help you rewire your brain. These experiments will give you amazing insights about your personality and state of mind, but they will also help you change and find out new transformational options in your life.

We will cover the importance of nourishing your body for increased activity in Chapter 8 in details. It is important to eat enough protein, which is the building block of muscles especially when you amp up your exercise regimen. Feel free to go there now if you are worried about your nutrition.

Let me now share the story of Daphne. I wish I could show you her picture but she is a very private person. She has been an inspiration to me. I have rarely found such a disciplined client. But it pays off!

Daphne's Story: How to Build Muscles at 70!

When Daphne (not her real name) came to see me the first time, she struck me as a person who would not need my help. She is not in this book about weight loss really. She is in this book because of her ability to transform her body. A much disciplined 73-year-old woman, Daphne is slim and elegant. Everything about her is beautiful: her white hair, her smooth complexion, her body shape and active mind. But she is one of those ladies who is not comfortable in her own skin if she weighs 135 pounds. She wanted to go back to 115 pounds, her "feel good" weight. Her extra 20 pounds made her feel fat—her own words. Everybody has a different perception of the perfect weight.

I have chosen Daphne as a story, because she was what I call a "skinny fat lady." Daphne discovered on my scales that she had 35% body fat, which made her very unhappy.

Daphne has a sweet tooth but only at the end of the day before going to bed. Although she rarely exceeded her BMR, except for the rare glass of wine or dessert, and ate very small portions, she needed to become smarter with food. She definitely did not eat enough protein, some days she was as low as 20 to 30g, when an average woman needs 50 to 60g. She stopped snacking before bed. We didn't need to cut her diet regimen, just chisel.

- We applied the carb+ fat+ protein principles
- She started to avoid starchy carbs after 4 p.m.
- She eliminated beans, which she loved, as a source of plant based protein and added more animal based protein
- She eliminated soups. Especially soups not homemade. They are full of unknown fats, starchy vegetables, rice or potatoes, and sugar when bought somewhere else.

She lost pounds by adhering to this new regimen, and of course increased her protein intake, some days adding a protein shake with vegetables in the afternoon after a workout. But there is so much you can do when a person is already a disciplined eater. She was not eating more than 1,000 to 1,200 calories a day. It was difficult to cut from that. We had to look at saving extra calories. We had to look at energy burning.

Yes, she wanted to lose 20 pounds at 73, and she was already exercising quite regularly. This is not an exercise-beginner story. But Daphne is not an exercise lover either. She is not an activity enthusiast. She is a discipline-driven person. I always say, motivation is nice, discipline is even better.

Daphne was in good shape in general. She was one of these "let's just get on the elliptical for 45 minutes at the same pace" type of girls. But that did not really help her lose weight!

I introduced her to interval training. She discussed it with her trainer who created a new routine for her. Daphne is very dedicated to her health and embarked on this new mission like a pro. This new push helped her in many ways. She also increased her strength training.
Her first Cogni-Shift was that she stopped being frustrated at not getting results fast enough. Secondly, she soon started to notice changes especially around her waist. Waist rolls were her number one complaint. No amount of activity could get rid of them. HIIT did it. She also started to allow herself more little treats once in a while without feeling guilty.

AT 75, DAPHNE HAS 25% BODY FAT! SHE LOST 10% POINTS!

In all honesty it took her more than one year. This is also a message I want to pass on. You need to be persistent and patient. Daphne is an inspiring story for several reasons. First is that it is never too late to exercise and build muscles. 75 is the new frontier! And second, there is so much you can cut in your diet…you do not want to live a life of deprivation, certainly not at 75! You want to have fun and joy in your life.

Moving is an essential marker of life longevity and quality, yes, but enjoying a nice meal with friends is also boosting your endorphins. Smart exercise, and building muscles, can either help you lose these last 5 stubborn pounds or just enjoy the perfect cupcake from time to time! Find your sweet spot. And enjoy the experiments this week. They may help you discover something you love.

....

This Week's Experiments

Experiment #1: Discover Your New Passion(s)

This one is simple. If you are already fit and accustomed to exercise, just either try a new activity you want to discover, add more cardio or strength in your weekly regimen or push yourself a little bit harder. If you are a beginner, start somewhere and challenge yourself a little bit more as your confidence and stamina increase. Also be curious, visit some gyms, discover some machines — there are so many new ones. Try some free classes, accompany a friend to a session, or think about what you liked to do when you were younger. Create your new resolutions with heart and gusto!

My New Resolution(s)	My Benefits
Example: I will add one more strength session to my week. I will splurge in a training session at my gym. I want to do learn how to exercise with TRX (it's suspension training where you use your own body as weight)	• I will build more muscles faster • I will burn more calories • I will be stronger • I have never done TRX, I may love it!
Example: I will start walking one hour every day, 4 days a week I will insert some high heart beat …..	• It will be good for my mood • I am curious to see the impact on my weight • Including intervals in my routine will make it more fun • I may also start to walk with ski poles
Insert Yours: (Try a new sport!)	

Experiment #2: Replace SATs with PATs and Move Your Butt!

This one will help you eliminate sabotaging thoughts. As you saw earlier, there is always a good excuse to not move. Remember that exercising does not have to do with going to the gym or getting on equipment or going running. It can be an increase in your activity level. Such as adding steps to your daily average by moving more at the office, at home etc. You can create opportunities to walk mire by parking your car further from your office, or when shopping. You can walk up more stairs. You can get a dog and start walking with it!

From SATs	To PATs and Actions!
Example: It's always too late to go to the gym. I don't have the courage to leave home anymore at the end of the day.	I will buy an elliptical machine and put it in front of the TV. They have very silent machines now. I can always find one on Craig's List! So no excuses anymore. **Or:** I will start booking a class at 6am, and get exercise out of the way.
Example: I am too fat and ugly to go to the gym. People will make fun of me.	I will start walking and follow cardio tapes at home to start. Once I have lost my first 10 lbs. I will splurge in a training session. I am going to the gym with my friend who has the same challenges. Together we are stronger I have nothing to be ashamed of. If I don't start at one point, I'll never change.
Write your own:	

Read your newly discovered PATs often, add some new ones, eliminate some once achieved or conquered. Write them in your diary and get inspired every day. Change occurs slowly but surely. Observe your body and mind evolve. You will note body changes in weeks and in days with HIIT!

Experiment #3: I Feel and Love the Change

This experiment will also help you retrain your brain to create new pleasure pathways as you start to enjoy a more active life. Some people on my program changed careers to become more active like Donna who decided to become a certified trainer. She discovered her love for fitness, and her even better defined body after losing 30 pounds. She realized she was an inspiration for people around her, and at her gym. People started to ask her to lead classes.

I don't want you to become a hamster on a wheel or get into robot mode. I just want for you to like, even love, doing it. And even if you can't get there yet, the best way is then to think how great you feel AFTER.

My Feelings and Observations:

- I feel calmer and content
- I noticed my mood improves when I run outside
- I love to be outside and enjoy nature
- I feel like a million bucks when I attend a spinning class
- I run faster now that I added strength training
- I sleep so much better
- I am more focused at work, I can also work for longer hours
- I have less sugar cravings
- I can play with my kids/grandkids etc.
- My knees don't hurt so much anymore
- Etc…

Experiment #4: Overcome Obstacles

INSTANT Cogni-Shift:

Have a flexible approach to exercising that allows you to listen to your body and mind needs. Just do what you can do, but do it!

Exercising when tired could lead to injury. If your head is not into it, you won't enjoy it either. What is important however is to have the discipline to adhere to your overall weekly plan, even if you missed one day!

I hear it often from non-exercisers who get over enthusiastic at first: "I will exercise five days a week". The chances are that the five times a week will become four or three some weeks because life gets in the way. But that is OK. Honestly once or twice a week as a goal is OK too especially for starters, but will you adhere to it? There are too many chances that something will pop up and sabotage your plans. You have to find your flow. But you also have to challenge yourself and stick to your self - commitment. This is why I always recommend splurging in a trainer, at least initially. He/she will give you good advice, and will gently push you week after week professionally. You do not want to get hurt.

So let's explore ways to motivate yourself to stick to your plan. What will you do, on these days where you have these terrible sabotaging thoughts, to get back on track? Learn what may be in your way from a practical point of view:

Examples of reasons why you may not feel like going exercising:

Reasons	Solutions
Fatigue vs. laziness	If really tired, maybe you exercised too much and have the weekend warrior syndrome. Take a rest for a few days If it's laziness, write down all the reasons why you want to lose weight and how exercise can help you. Also think about how great you will feel after. Reflect on the progress so far, it will encourage you.

Reasons	Solutions
Not liking the exercise or activity vs. liking it (are you really doing something you like?)	Have you really looked at new options or new activities? Have you challenged your trainer to become more creative (maybe time to find another one)?
Not seeing results quickly enough and getting discouraged too easily	Speak with your trainer or somebody at the gym. Have you taken your body measures before and after? Some gyms even offer this service for free. They even may have a body composition machine or manual caliper. Maybe you are a little bit too impatient? Or are you pushing yourself hard enough?
Exercising too much, while not eating enough, which gets you into a real state of constant fatigue – and usually lack of weight loss	This is a syndrome I have seen often. You have to go back to Chapter 5 and look at your minimal calorie intake for weight loss/BMR while exercising. If you burn an extra 500 calories a day exercising while depriving your body of food, your body will hold on to its fat reserves.
Same old routine every day?	Vary the machines, classes, types of exercises. Mix and match different routines. Discover something new.
Being in real pain vs. workout after burn?	This is a tricky one. We all may endure pain after a heavy strength session especially if we have not trained for a while. It is due to the build-up of lactic acid in our muscles. To get rid of the pain, it's recommended to move. Go back to the gym and train in a gentler way, like running if you had a tough body building session the day before. Monitor your body for unusual aches. Don't ignore them. Check with your doctor if the pain is unusual or persists.

This is the end of what I would like you to accomplish in the coming weeks. All these experiments do not have to be conducted in one week. This is part of your journey. I want you to become more attuned with your body and mind reinvention. Don't overdo it and injure yourself.

Cogni-Tip:

This chapter's experiments could be done over a couple of weeks especially if you are a beginner. You will need a few weeks, 4 to 6 in fact, to start to see results. Well done HIIT exercises on the other hand will show results even after one week.

CogniDiet® Book Club Discussion Guide

This week, it's all about your body and your muscles! It's time, if not done yet, to find a partner in your book club or elsewhere and start an exercising group. It really makes a difference to have a buddy! Working out together fosters encouragement, healthy competition and motivation.

You are not always going to be motivated. But you will get results by getting disciplined. Please make sure you take pictures weekly to document your transformation.

- **Does everybody exercise in the group? If yes, share how you amped up the efforts, started HIIT, a new routine or new sport.**

- **If some of you do not exercise, don't like to exercise (even walking is a stretch LOL), or have a hard time exercising due to health and physical problems, how is the group going to help them get started?**

- **What are your biggest obstacles? Ask the group to help you overcome them.**

- **If there is an exercise champion in the group, can she share pictures before and after, how she transformed her body, how she feels after exercise etc.?**

- **How are you all going to integrate exercise within this next 5 weeks? Share your commitment. Share some new goals. Be serious about it.**

- **Is there a way you can make exercise more fun?**

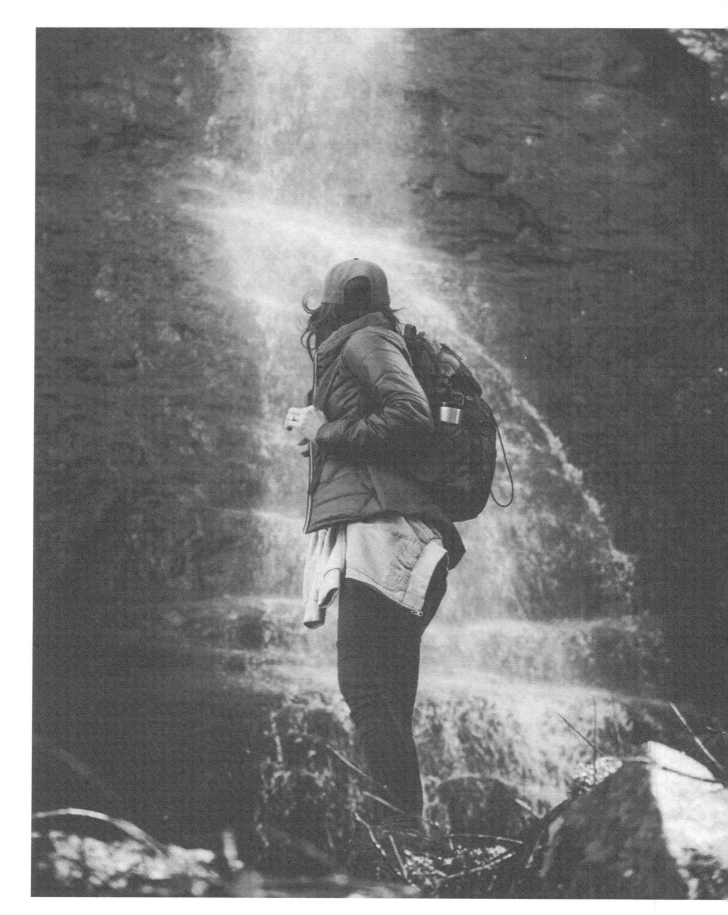

Part 2
The Next 6 Weeks

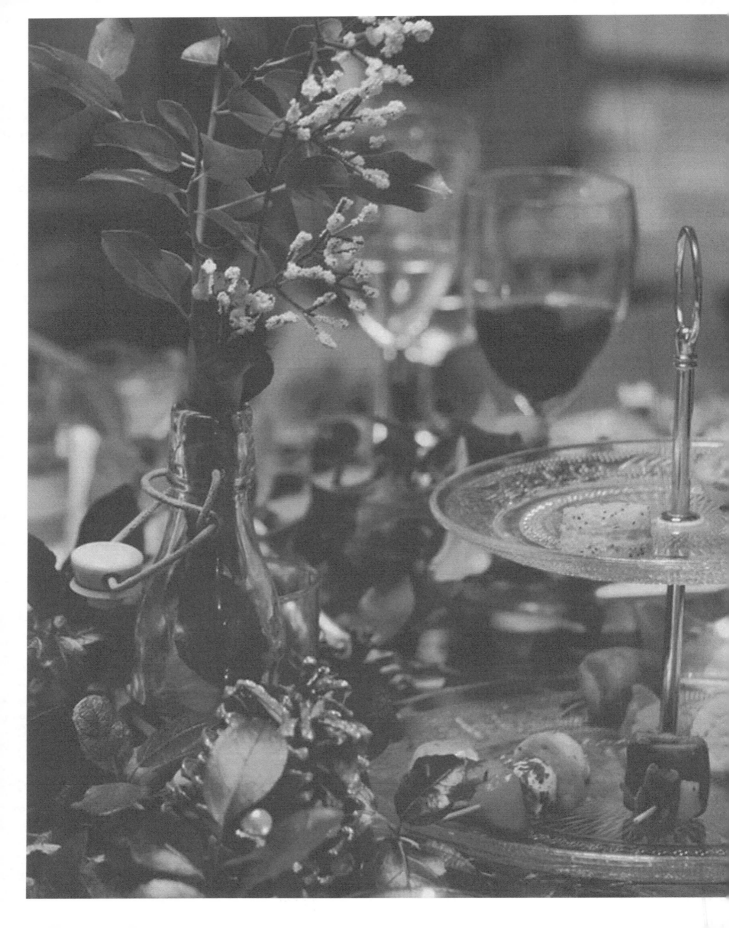

Chapter 7

I Deal With Saboteurs and Eat Mindfully

Nobody and Nothing Can Own My Brain

In this chapter you will learn to deal with saboteurs, including yourself. They can be well intentioned. Knowing what your needs are, what your hunger level is and being mindful about the moment are key to deal with these situations. We will start with the saboteurs and then help you get more attuned to your hunger level. Being more mindful in your decisions and actions, and feeling what you need rather than what you want is key to overcoming these sabotaging situations.

Aaaaah, how can you resist true love? How can you say no to a slice of cake, when you feel deep inside, that you are going to hurt someone's feelings or look impolite? What if there is some form of gentle, yet real, bullying in being offered yet another slice of this delicious home-made pie? Because it was baked with love, just for you, the way you liked it as a kid. And to make it even more challenging, what if it was baked or bought by your own very loving mother? The mother whom you are visiting will say "I just went to that special bakery—took me an hour to get there (hello guilt!)—to buy these delicious chocolate frosted cupcakes you loved as a kid. I had them specially ordered for you (even more guilt if you refuse one). Have one, it won't hurt, please don't tell me you are on a diet, yet again." What do you do when food is associated with love, and receiving it is so important to the giver? And frankly, what are the real motives behind the food pushing and its acceptance? You will say love on both sides, but what else?

The Sacred Sisterhood Evening Club

How many times have you gone out with girlfriends to enjoy drinks and a nice meal and share the sacred sisterhood's secrets and wonderful camaraderie? There is always the skinny one, so annoyingly perfect who can eat and drink whatever she wants. And yes, she will push you to have another cocktail, treating you like a party pooper if you don't. She will say: "Nora is on a diet again. You're no fun Nora, come on girl, we see each other's only four times a year and you have chosen that day to become a teetotaler? Hmm, I remember you not so long ago! Hello margaritas plural." "Yes, tough, I've changed," you mumble under your breath. How will you say no and yet keep the spirit of the party?

The Dessert Sharer

Or the other girlfriend, the one who manages her own guilt by ordering desserts "to share", so she is not just on her own having one. This way she won't feel so bad. How will you resist the scrumptious caramel fudge ice cream when a spoon is placed in your hand? She will say, "Let's be good tomorrow, we only live once, this dessert is only made in this restaurant with a secret recipe to die for, it's only a bite, let's enjoy it together".

"You're a Debbie downer, start your diet tomorrow, it's only for today, go with the flow, you just can't have fun anymore, why don't you eat—isn't it good? Are you unhappy, is something wrong?"

How many times have you heard these remarks as you valiantly try to follow your own healthy routine? This happens in a social context most of the times, but the danger can loom at home every day with a couple of in-house saboteurs.

The Sugar-Loving Family Member

On the other hand, I have so many positive stories, about clients with supportive partners or family members. The "mamma" who will cook specifically for her daughter in order to support her weight loss. The husband who is eating his ice cream in his office, not with his wife, or in front of the TV anymore. The wife who banished pretzels from the household so her husband would stop eating them.

In those situations it often came down to my clients having the courage to just ask them to make an effort and be respectful of their journey. And in 90% of the cases, the support occurred. Don't use a potential hypothetical refusal as a pre-emptive sabotaging thought though. Be assertive in your needs.

You Can Be Your Own Best Own Saboteur

On the other hand, I bet you have a saboteur in the family that may be very close to you. She is your shadow, your nemesis, your Mr. Hyde. And you encounter sabotaging situations often together. Some of you will say they live in a permanent state of sabotage. You may have a hard time facing parties, because she follows you. She stalks you. Especially when alcohol is present, or when the office meeting room presents these awful—cheap, bad quality—cookies every afternoon. You hear her little voice, full of SATs in your head. So many excuses! What about the ice cream parlor every summer while spending time at the beach? You know the one I am talking about! The one ice cream parlor with the special multicolored colossal cone. The kids have it every day after 6 hours of running and swimming at the beach, while you were Facebooking and reading a novel. Yes, but you have to have it too because this is part of Mr. Hyde's daily vacation ritual...

And do you recognize yourself here as "the loving baker"? What better excuse than baking for others. It is an act of love and can be a lifelong hobby. But how many times do you lick the batter? How many cookies did you eat, in between batches? How many scrumptious desserts did you whip for your family? If you have a sweet tooth, I recommend you find a new hobby!

We hope at this stage of the program that you have developed your own Cogni-Shifts to fight yourself?

The Food Industry is Manipulating Your Brain and Taste Buds

In reality, every moment of the day can become a self-sabotaging act to your own efforts. Life is littered with tempting people and occasions. Just watching TV is a big non-stop production of commercials all targeting your senses and emotions, from orgasm-triggering mint flavored cookies to psychedelic dream-inducing potato chips. How many coffee shops can there be in a bloc in New York? You are tempted at every corner, by the same chain.

Analyze the TV and magazine food ads in the coming weeks. Find out the subliminal messages. Observe the words used, the images, and the lyrics and/or music. The food and beverage industries are spending billions of dollars every year to manipulate your brain. If they do it, and it works, you must be able to resist and rewire your brain the other way around. They have food engineers, flavor researchers, and color artists. They travel the world for new tastes. They even test food colors with consumers. They know sugar-fat ratios to a T, because this mixture is the most pleasurable taste bud sensation. The food is fizzing. The candies are exploding. The chocolate is melting in layers.

Going on a diet requires controlling the food and the situation at every moment. This means not watching TV, shopping for healthy food, cooking and eating at home, avoiding or planning visits, parties and restaurants. But who can live like this?

Are we doomed with weight loss, and condemned to a life of isolation and deprivation? We may as well stay on a desert island. Of course, my answer is no and I will share some tools to help you be more in control and more mindful about how and when to eat. The problem is we let the environment control us versus us staying on top of what we really want. I mean, what you want, not what the food industry wants you to want, to crave, to desire, to long for.

But control and willpower can only last so long. At one point you will falter, let loose and get totally out of control. It's like a dam that breaks. All the emotions and self-deprivation that have been contained are unleashed all of a sudden. The cravings are super-powered as the brain has been in a state of penance for too long. Remember, your brain wants pleasure.

Besides your goals, and visualization and calming techniques mentioned earlier, you will learn in this chapter to become more aware and mindful about your food choices. The more mindful you are about your hunger and own needs, the more you will find it natural and easier to just say "no, thank you".

A Word of Encouragement – Never Give up!

This has been my path, this has been my fight. Everything I mentioned earlier, except the sabotaging husband, I lived. I have been knocked down by a Twizzlers® attack (my weakness) more than once even since I became healthier. I have caved in again to a Boston crème doughnut not so long ago. I have emptied a bucket of ice cream once in a while. I have said "f...k this life style" to myself. I have cried. I have looked at myself in the mirror not liking my fat rolls. I have witnessed my scale going up—by 4 pounds in two days! I have been jealous of my skinny friends. I have seen my hemoglobin A1c level rise. I have noticed my puffy face after a carb-rich meal. I have felt like a failure. But I have not dieted for the past 10 years. How do I succeed?

 Cogni-Tip:

Persevere, persevere, girlfriend. Never give up!

I persevere. I never give up. I put my tangible goals and benefits ahead of a taste of something. I question myself. I stop in my tracks. I often laugh, gently, at myself. Years ago, I started eliminating one danger after the other. My dangers are not yours. We all are different. But sugar is a common thread, even bigger than portion issues. It is an addiction. I became aware of what sugar and carbs were triggering in my body years ago. I began to dissect the disintegration of foods in my body with the eyes of a chemist. I faced what extra sugar in my blood was doing to my organs. I worked in diabetes in big pharma. First I stopped eating pasta, then pizza, and then bread at lunch or dinner. Guess, what, I do not miss them. But I have pasta or pizza once in a while, — good ones and in small portions.

Then I looked at my Twizzlers® label and it sank in that I was eating pure chemicals. I have kept doughnuts from a famous food chain at the office – in a sort of shrine, for all to witness. They have been there since November 2013. Still smelling and looking darn good in 2017. Just a little bit dehydrated and tough, with a few visible sugar crystals on the surface! I bet I could eat them and not die, yet.

I led the CogniDiet® curriculum classes so many times, that I positively brainwashed myself. I installed MyFitnessPal® on my iPhone®, I cut portions, I started HIIT. I fell of the wagon, I got back on the saddle. And I am not a party pooper. I am just firm, yet discreet. I snack on nuts. I won my battle one pound at a time. I just learned to not compromise anymore, with grace. This has been going on for 10 years. I have been victorious for 10 years. I am mindful of my needs and wants.

I say to myself: "This is not good enough for me!"

I know my body. I know what works or not, what is nutritional and pleasurable versus dangerous and pleasurable. You can too if you decide to love your body and health more than a Snickers Bar®.

Write your warrior princess motto. The one when you feel slapping yourself in the face because you are facing this unfair warm and crusty croissant at a breakfast meeting. Your wake up call, your fighting motto, your "let's get over this once and for all" shout:

- I'm done with you
- F...k this bagel
- It's over diet soda (as if you were breaking up with somebody)
- I'm not your friend anymore (I mean you are dumping your old bestie peanut butter cream cupcake)
- Not my cup of tea anymore

What is your warrior cry my friends? Write it NOW – and then just shout it loudly, just for the fun of it:

My Warrior Cry!

Once this is out of your system, and you feel better about it, just inhale, take a moment to enjoy this liberating moment and think about how free you are. Talking, crying, shouting, writing, sharing and even maybe drawing your resolve and self- healing actions is part of the process of change. I like a good kick in the butt moment from time to time. And then I re-center myself around my balance and serenity.

You got in control with your warrior mind. Now is time to become mindful again. And consider the results of your – good – decision. You expelled the negative energy. Now enjoy your calm.

INSTANT Cogni-Shift:

There is **CONTROL** and there is **MINDFULNESS.** Mindfulness is when you are **ONE** with your body and brain. There are no reins needed. Saboteurs can't reach you. You are free.

What are Your Worst Sabotaging Situations?

Let's first deal with saboteurs and sabotaging situations and then see how you can handle them gently but firmly. I always say that NOBODY can force you to put anything in your mouth unless you decide to. Even a loving mother. This is a fundamental human right come to think about it. I love Judy Orloff's book "Positive Energy". I recommend it to many clients who need to deal with too much stress. In this book, she teaches you to shield against "energy vampires".

INSTANT Cogni-Shift:

The technique is to surround yourself with an invisible positive mental protective shield. I use this technique when I feel I am in a food danger zone. I cloak myself, if I decide to, and pass through the temptation unscathed. It is a powerful technique.

So let's find out your most vulnerable moments and sabotaging situations and learn to deal with them first.

What are they mostly related to?

- Travel
- Certain people
- Social and family events
- Stress
- Being happy, or being unhappy
- Boredom
- Rituals
- Shopping
- Restaurants and bars
- Vacation time
- Holiday season
- Work and meetings
- All of the above?

Now, Let's Deal With These Sabotaging Situations. What Type of Personality Are You?

Now let's find ways to deal with these situations. You can decide what type of personality you are or will become. Be in charge. Be centered on your needs. Don't let yourself be bullied. Remember that avoidance is a very powerful strategy. If you have a weakness for finger foods and cocktails, why are you such a social butterfly going from party to party? Maybe there is a compromise there? Please role-play after having selected your worst saboteurs. And don't be afraid to wear multiple personalities. Your goal requires some smart strategies and you are authorized a few white lies!

Personality #1: The assertive

The answer/action: "Thank you Mom, I love you, but I cannot eat these cookies anymore with my pre-diabetes. I appreciate this loving gesture. I will bring them with me and give them to/please Mom here are a few recipes of authorized baked goods for me, maybe we could learn to cook them together."

If a friend wants to serve you a third time with her home baked lasagna, just have the courage to say "no thank you, I am full."

The assertive people just stand up for themselves. They will make their goals and needs clear to everybody, including their loved ones.

Personality #2: The diplomat

The answer/action: "This looks dangerously delicious. I'll pass but will have a small bite just for you (or I will take some home)!"

These people usually conform to the environment but minimize its impact in a gracious way. They are a little bit manipulative!

Personality #3: The avoider

The answer/action: "Sorry, can't get to the party tonight."

Start to look at your agenda and eliminate the too many dinners, parties penciled in. You do not need to be out and about every night of the week.

If you do need to be out too frequently, for your job, you may have to consider other strategies. A white lie does not hurt once in a while (headache, family, conference call, etc.)

Personality #4: The white liar

The answer/action: "Thank you Caroline, I am avoiding gluten now (not a real lie)." "I am not feeling too well, I have to be careful with food today".

It looks like enough information and usually people will not dare to ask indiscreet questions, nor push you to eat more.

Personality #5: The schemer

The answer/action: To be transparent, I have been that one, more than once. I have taken that awful office birthday cake from the kitchen, where I had a bite, and then under the guise of going back to work, thrown the remainder in my trash can.

I also know some women who are very good at pretending they are eating. They just play with their food. Or they keep a plate full during the entire cocktail party!

Personality #6: The planner

The answer/action: Bring your own food, carry your survival pack (for me it is nuts), eat before the party, allow yourself a food and drink budget for the night, scan the buffet, check menus before selecting a restaurant etc.

This person wants to participate, while staying in control. Planning is time consuming! It may require research. But it is a very successful strategy. Just the planning in itself is rewiring your brain.

What is your style?

Write down some of your future strategies. You can mix and match different roles!

Now think about your most predictable scenarios and challenges, and get ready. If you feel that the problem is not that you can't say NO, but that in reality you love, adore, can't resist the drink, the cookie or the extra lasagna serving, then we have to come up with other solutions.

Remember, you can select from what you learned, and practiced in this book so far:

- Go back to your goals and benefits. What matters to you most?
- Remember your vision board?
- What have you accomplished so far? Be proud about your victories. You may have lost 10 pounds or more by now!
- Visualize your new you
- Utilize the emotional brain technique to summon an image that will make your brain happy vs. a piece of chocolate
- Breathe slowly and deeply
- Practice your distractions list
- What about your PATs?
- Have you spoken to your saboteurs and outlined your needs?

Cogni-Game:

Practice your personality. Prepare answers and excuses BEFORE you get into the situation. Or just avoid them.

Besides avoidance of a situation, which is not always possible, become more open, even honest, about your own issues. The tough situations can trigger emotions from the past, souvenirs that can be both comforting and soothing to you. Souvenirs can also be painful and food is used as a way to deal with it. A mother can get you back in a child-like state of obedience—and yes, fear—even if you are 60 years old! If nothing has worked so far, maybe this book is not for you, and I'm sorry about it. But in my heart I believe that change is the only way to go. Maybe close the book, take a break. Think about your motivation to change (remember) and see if you moved the needle along.

There are also all the underlying currents present with friends, family or colleagues interactions, such as the need to conform to society and go with the flow. As humans we want to feel accepted and liked. Especially when your boss is involved! Some of us are more assertive than others - I am - of their needs and strict about their resolutions. You can still be gracious but firm about them. You can also be discreet. You do not have to trumpet across the whole table that you will not have bread with olive oil. In fact, based on years of experience, I can tell you how little people will pay attention, in a group, to what you eat or drink. Just pretend to follow the flow.

Cogni-Tip:

Follow the flow but still manage your owns needs. Stay in control. Here are a few tricks I've learned over the years:

- Seat at the end of a table when with a group, less attention will be placed on your drinks or plate
- Carry a full plate or drink with you at party, but don't touch it. People will leave you alone
- Don't say anything about your weight or health goals, people may tease you and provoke you
- Drink and eat slowly, people, again, won't notice
- Always scan a buffet, then make your choices, then put what you chose on your plate. Do not discover the offerings haphazardly following the buffet flow, you will end up putting too much on your plate
- Bring your own healthy food to a party
- Drink spritzers or "fake" cocktails
- Don't approach the food table at a party, you won't be tempted. Embark in lively conversations or activities
- Negotiate the menu, when you can, before a family or friends party, if you can. With my family I ask them to cook things I like, and that are healthy

- Move the meeting cookie tray from the middle of the table to a side table
- Focus on people, conversations, activities, not food
- Ignore the saboteurs, avoid them. Wear your protective bad energy shield!

These are strategies for managing these never ending temptations. But the best technique, the one that has really helped most of my clients at the end, is to be mindful of their hunger level. And this one is also the best at fighting your self-sabotaging behaviors.

Your Hunger Level – Are You Aware of It?

Some of us can be wavering, following the mood of the moment. There is not one recipe. But awareness about your real hunger is not questionable, it is a survival skill.

Cogni-Tip:

We must eat to live, but we must eat right, and only when needed frankly, to live well. Make it your new motto.

I always hear from clients who follow the 12-week program that becoming aware of their hunger level and following its guidance was the most important skill they acquired. If you are MINDFUL, there is not ONE saboteur that can get at you, promised!

Cogni-Tip:

If you are not hungry when that food is getting close to your mouth, you are not eating mindfully!

Let's Play the Hunger Games

Most of us have become disconnected from our real hunger level. We are constantly pushing something, including as a liquid, in our throats. Walk in a city and observe what people are carrying in the streets. One out of three person will have a drink or some kind of food in his/her hands. Eating has become a day-long hobby.

There are 10 levels of hunger, ranging from starving at Level One to being completely over-stuffed and bursting from food after a feast of gluttony at Level 10!

The Hunger Meter, The 10 Hunger Levels:

1. Famished: Stomach completely empty, weak, light headed

2. Starving: Feeling uncomfortable, irritable, unable to concentrate

3. Uncomfortably Hungry: Stomach is rumbling

4. Slightly Hungry: Just starting to feel hunger

5. Neutral: Satisfied

6. Satisfied: Just ate the right amount of food

7. Completely Satisfied: A bit too full. You know you do not need that extra bite anymore!

8. Uncomfortably Full: Bloated, uneasy

9. Very Uncomfortable: Clothes are too tight, feel like a balloon

10. Stuffed: Need stomach relief, want to sleep. Could be sick

Most of the time, between meals, we should be at the neutral level, or at Level Five. Pause now for a few seconds and gauge your current hunger level. How are you feeling? If at Level Five, there is no reason to reach to that little snack next to your book, right?

It's important to measure your hunger level frequently. This way you learn to become more aware of your needs. When was it that you really, really, felt like starving? You were ravenous and would have eaten anything presented to you. But in our society, here in the U.S., unless you are at poverty level, when are you seriously starving? The only time I can remember being in that state is as a kid, after a whole afternoon of non-stop strenuous physical activity. The dinner could not come soon enough. I would not even call it Level 1. We were just ravenous. Or maybe after a long run a few years ago.

On the other hand, once you start eating, you should try to never exceed Level 6 or 7. Level 6 is perfect because it is when you just know it's enough. You are completely satisfied. You do not need that extra bite anymore. You know you don't.

Remember these never-ending Thanksgiving dinners with the coma inducing sweetness, from the cranberry jelly to the marshmallow sprinkled sweet potato pie. And the eggnog, and the wine, and the macaroni gratin. How do you feel at the end of the dinner? How much of this food is really delicious and nourishing? When do you reach Level 8? Is it worth your while? Have you ever been sick after such a dinner? I have.

Your stomach, when empty, is the size of one closed fist, maybe two fists for bigger persons or eaters. The more you eat, the stretchier the stomach will become. This is why people undergoing stomach-reducing or stapling surgery can, after a few years, re-stretch their stomach and eat a lot again.

Cogni-Game:

I know it's not very appetizing, but imagine your empty stomach before you eat as you face your plate or meal. Try to gauge the food volume on your plate and how it will make your stomach stretch. More than once, this mental exercise made me cut my portions.

The more you get attuned and in sync with your real appetite, the less you will eat. The awareness goes both ways: when are you hungry and when are you satiated? It is crucial to become really aware at that and then decide if you still want to eat this dessert after a large meal!

There are however a few tricks to eat less, of the bad stuff:

- Drink a glass of water before the meal and drink more water in general
- Eat a salad, or vegetables first, they will occupy more volume in your stomach especially if they are high in fiber/water
- Eating more slowly and more mindfully (one later experiment is about that)
- Have protein rich snacks. They take more time to be digested and will help you keep hunger at bay
- Have fiber rich foods such as chia or flax seeds for breakfast. Again being rich in soluble fiber, they will occupy space in your stomach!

Trisha's Story: My Husband is My Biggest Saboteur

I decided today to share a story that is bitter sweet. The reason I am sharing it is for those of you who are stuck in a not so happy situation. It can be related to a job, a relationship, or a family situation. You are in fact dealing with an energy vampire. You have to fight constantly for your priorities.

I'll always remember this lovely client whose skinny husband was a sugar addict. Trisha is not her real name. He did not take it well that she had decided to forgo sugar. In a form of vengeance or rebellion, because he felt guilty he wasn't, he started to buy more and more of the forbidden foods, and planted them all over the house. She has two kids and the standard diet at home was pretty regular hamburgers, barbecues with few vegetables, macaroni and cheese, Chinese take-outs and sodas. It has not been easy to get the family more health conscious either.

Her husband was testing her resolve. You know what I am talking about. He wants you skinny and constantly belittles you for your weight and looks, yet sabotages all your efforts. It is called bullying.

Not a very supporting husband will you say, but a real situation. He even refused to stash his treasure in a special cupboard so she would not be tempted by it. He refused to stop eating his treats while they were watching TV. Imagine her pain while she was trying to stick to sugar-free yogurt with fresh strawberries while her husband was crunching Kit-Kats® with great pleasure next to her. The chocolate aroma was titillating her nose, making it impossible to resist. Then he would get an ice cream - vanilla and cookie dough - on a cone.

The torture was nonstop. Sometimes, in a moment of weakness, when all her willpower and PATs and visualization tricks had failed, she would go in the kitchen and have a secret ice cream lick directly from the bucket in the freezer. Or, she just caved in and took the bucket. Then came the guilt, the sense of failure and this horrible feeling that life is not fair in so many ways. She cried in front of me many times.

I have to stay she struggled and did not really manage to lose significant weight, only a few pounds at the end. She yo-yoed during the 12 week program. She had good weeks, interestingly when her husband was traveling. Her house was a sugar booby trap when he was back home.

After multiple strategic attempts at tackling the issue, she finally started a plan. She decided to be more assertive. But she took all the initiatives. For a while it worked, and this is why I want to share this story with you today.

- She stopped watching TV with him and went reading instead, in her bedroom. Reading also calmed her down after a busy day
- She started to systematically put his sugary stuff back in a special cupboard. He was unhappy with it, but learned to deal with it, for a while
- Her other tactic was she gave him a big box or container that sat on the kitchen counter, containing his stash. The lid was dark. This way, the candies weren't visible to her eyes.
- She put the ice cream in the garage freezer and not in the kitchen one. This made it more challenging for her to get to the ice cream source
- She walked every evening after dinner, in order to stay away from temptations and burn more calories
- She enrolled her kids in the "hiding" effort. They supported her.

He finally got the message, more or less. But this guy to this day is still not supporting her 100%. This story is particularly cruel because she was really trying hard.

What would you have done differently? My advice to her was to stay the course and start to look at these sugary temptations with a new eye like Sharon. And tame that darn husband of hers!

....

This Week's Experiments

Experiment #1: Eat mindfully

Next time you have lunch or dinner, do the following:

- Measure your appetite level to start with
- Assess what you will need, based on this assessment, and on what you know will be served. This gives you control. You may even start the meal by sharing your appetite level with the cook or host in a polite manner — so that they don't serve you a gigantic portion!
- As you eat, try to slow down, chew more than usual, something better done initially on your own as an experiment!
- Put your fork and knife back on the table after each morsel. This is another way to slow down
- Become more interested in savoring the food and assessing the flavors, textures, colors on your plate and in your palate. Use all your senses. Again, this will slow you down. You can also express compliments to the host/cook that are well turned!
- Try to elongate your meal as much as you can and become aware about how long it took for a standard two course meal (starter and main course, or main course and dessert)

Now, in your diary, and in retrospect, how quickly have you eaten last time you had a meal — not the experiment mentioned above? Do you remember? I bet it could be as fast as 10 minutes. If you shove food very quickly into your mouth, and don't chew it long enough, not only is it not good for your digestion, but it will fill your stomach too quickly. There will be no real pleasure in the meal, come to think about it. The goal of this experiment is to make you think twice before you put food next time in your mouth, especially in a sabotaging situation.

Ask yourself the following questions:

- Am I hungry?
- Do I need this? Is this making me happy and content, really?
- Is this food good enough for me, my body and my mind?
- Is this food necessary to help me enjoy this very moment
- What is the quality of this food, what are the ingredients?
- Would I prepare this myself, would I eat this (crap) at home?
- Is this food worthwhile, because of its deliciousness, to make me veer from my resolutions?
- Will I regret not eating it? Really?

Experiment #2: Eat in 20 minutes minimum

Next meal, if you can, with your family or on your own, put a timer on the table and eat in at least 20 minutes. I mean a two course meal.

Cogni-Tip:

It takes 20 minutes to your stomach to tell your brain it is full.

After the meal, note your impressions and feelings in your diary, or discuss it with the family. It is a good experience for all around the table, including kids. They may make fun of you, but I did this at home, including when I was hosting cooking classes and participants had many insights. They discovered:

- When eating more slowly, they ate less
- When they started the meal with high fiber content food, like mixed vegetables or salads, their stomach filled in with "bigger volume" foods first and they ate much less of the starchy carbs and protein later, and had no room left for desserts!

- Chewing more often is kind of "tiring", it slows you down and forces you to stay focused on your mouth rather than your food.
- One day we even organized a blinded dinner. The guests' eyes were covered with one of those airplanes sleeping masks. My husband and I had cooked a secret meal. The guests had to guess what they were eating, what spices and herbs were used etc. Yes, it was challenging to find the food served on the pate, so that slowed the eating process down. But the biggest aha moment was how little they had eaten. Their eyes were not there to fool them with portion sizes. They ate totally in accordance with their appetite. The conversation was sparse, maybe due to the concentration needed for eating! Quasi silence also fostered more mindfulness I bet.

Then on the other hand, eat the same menu very quickly one other day, in let's say 10 minutes, and see how you feel about your hunger. The goal of these two experiments is to teach you to eat more slowly, therefore eat less!

Experiment #3: Play the hunger game — Only if your health permits

The more you are attuned to your hunger the more you become what we call a "natural eater". In fact, natural eaters may not be in need to have a well-orchestrated breakfast, lunch and dinner regimen. They may end up skipping meals because that day they weren't so active, therefore not hungry. Our society, and rituals have created the three meals a day tradition. However our ancestors just ate when they could and when they needed it. Your body is still engineered this way.

This experiment is to help you to get more attuned to your REAL hunger. Select a day. Go as long as you can, with not eating, if your health permits. Try to get yourself at Level four or five of real hunger. Preferably skip a breakfast or lunch, or both.

Note how you feel as the day goes by. Again, I do not want you to end up in a state of hypoglycemia, but you will realize that you can really go a long way without being in need of food. Describe your hunger symptoms. Is it a headache, being grumpy, becoming unable to focus, stomach rumblings?

Experiment #4: Eating seated, eating and just eating

Are you always seated when eating? How many times have you caught yourself walking while biting on that sandwich between two meetings or munching on a cookie between the kitchen and the family room? And mothers who cook and eat while, before and after the meal is served? Finishing the kids' plates? Is that familiar?

When seated, your brain associates this position with eating. You are in the moment. Of course, not while being on Facebook.

While walking, reading, or working on your computer, your brain engages in other distracting activities, which separate you from the act of eating. Do you really think you are enjoying and registering that hotdog you eat while walking in NYC? You are not attuned to your hunger at that moment. You will eat mindlessly. You may even over eat, remember the 20min rule. You are not savoring the meal. You are rushing. You are not giving your body the attention and care it deserves.

When in corporate America, and maybe these are my French roots, I really always tried to take a break for lunch and go to the cafeteria or out to buy something. And eating while just doing that. I even noticed than when doing that, I was not touching the cookies at the 2 p.m. meeting.

This week observe yourself, at least for one day. Don't even take one bite while not seated. You will notice, it is very hard!

Cocktail party will you say? Yes they are an exception. But even at these parties, there is often a seated section or at least standing tables. In that case, at least check your hunger level!

Experiment #5: Eat one — or several — of your temptations mindfully. Yes, you can!

Yes, this one experiment has scared more than one client. In fact I did it myself with my famous Twizzlers®. I also did it with "dulce de leche" ice cream, one of my favorites. This is how I decided never to have a Twizzlers® in my life anymore. I realized the taste was not so fantastic and the ingredients were crap. This is also how I realized how sugary ice cream is — and it had consequences. I allow myself an ice cream a month, and it has to be the best one. I also take a reasonable portion. I savor it.

Select one of your favorite go to temptation food. The one you know is sabotaging your weight loss attempts. The delicious little sinful secret. The life-long addiction. The comfort food. The one thing that will make you get up at 9 p.m., and go to the store just to buy it! You don't have to do this with one temptation. You can do the experiment with several. I bet it's not roasted zucchinis.

The goal is to make you more mindful about eating it and disassociating it from emotions. Eating it as an experiment will force you to use more of your logical and fact based left brain. You are like a detective, analyzing a situation.

Here is the hit-parade of the top ones I heard over the years:

- Ice cream
- Chips or pretzels – something salty and crunchy
- Warm fresh bread
- Chocolate
- Specific sweets
- Ice cream
- Pizza
- What is yours – can be plural!

Take your temptation food, sit down and start to eat it mindfully. Make it a ceremonial. Eat it slowly. Notice the flavors, textures. Take your time. Find out what makes it so pleasurable. Some of you told me they were afraid the experiment would trigger a vicious cycle. If it does, then you really know it is a dangerous food and needs to disappear from your menu.

After you've eaten it. Take your diary and note all that you really like, and don't like, about it. Maybe you will discover it's not so good after all.

Read the label, find the ingredients. Digest the information. Think about what these ingredients do your body. If it's a name you don't understand, Google it. Discover the amount of sugar (4g is one teaspoon) you just ate. If it's carbohydrates, translate the grams of carbohydrates into sugar.

Three outcomes are possible after the experiment:

1. You don't like it so much, after all. Then, get rid of it once and for all. If you still have some at home, throw it away.

2. You really love it. Then make a deal with yourself, unless it triggers uncontrolled cravings. Have it once a week, or once a month for instance. Never when stressed out. Only when you decide it, and savor it.

3. Find a substitute if it is really dangerous. For me less than 70% cocoa content in chocolate is too sugary and triggers unstoppable cravings. 85% chocolate will make me content with just one square (50 calories). This shows how sensitive I am to sugar.

To conclude this chapter, which again, is a very important one, take a break, close your eyes and decode your own current behaviors. At this juncture, you must have had many aha moments already. You must have surprised yourself. Usually after 7 weeks on the program, the body and mind transformations are very visible. There is a feeling of joy and a lot of energy in the class. I always ask participants to go around the table and list all of their accomplishments so far. A victory, does not have to be a pound lost. Having cooked your first home made meal is a major reason to celebrate. Having shopped for the first time for a gym and getting to a yoga class can be a revolution at 65! Having said no to second servings and a loving saboteur is quite an accomplishment!

To conclude this chapter, I am asking YOU to write all of your achievements so far, small and big, health, weight, and stress related. And I am sending you a big loving hug across your shrinking body and expanding confidence!

MY FREAKINGLY IMPRESSIVE ACHIEVEMENTS!

_____

_____

_____

_____

_____

_____

_____

_____

_____

_____

CogniDiet® Book Club Discussion Guide

This week is all about managing saboteurs and using mindfulness to become more attuned to your real hunger level. You will have a lot to share with your group. I recommend that for fun you organize a blindfolded meal together. You will need an accomplice to be the cook, a server and to keep everything a secret! Or you can share a mindful meal together and discuss your findings and feelings.

- **Do you have saboteurs in your life? Ask your friends to help you manage them**
- **Role-play on how to navigate a tough situation.**
- **Did you gauge your hunger level (most important experiment)? What did you learn from it?**
- **Have you tested some of your biggest temptations and eaten them mindfully?**
- **What did you observe when you ate in 20 minutes? Or in less?**
- **Share your impressive list of achievements!**

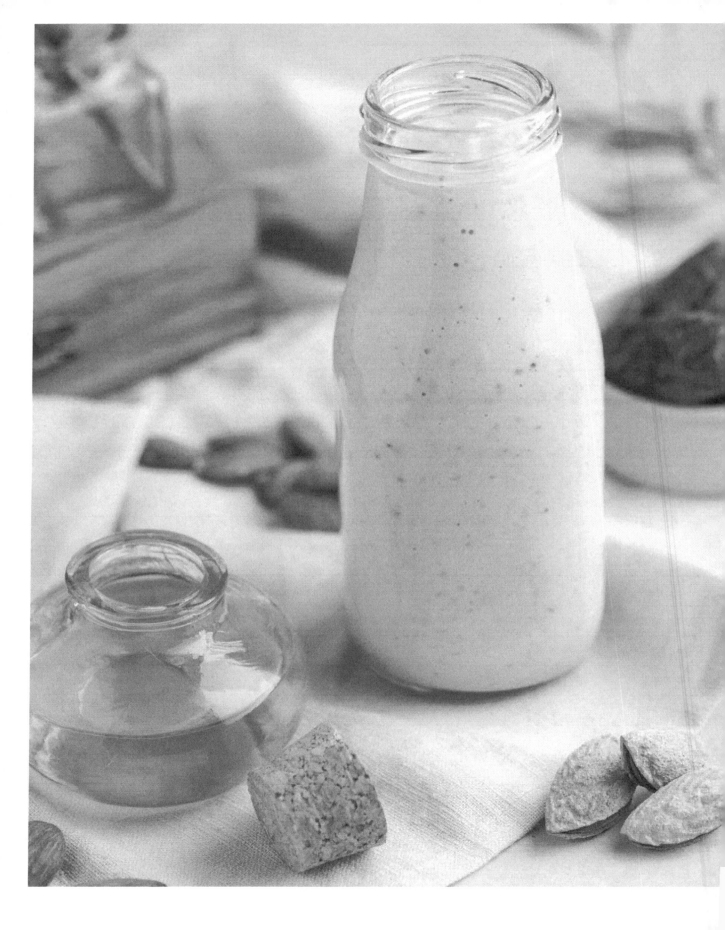

Chapter 8

Friendly Fat and Powerful Protein — Yes, They Can Help Me Lose Weight!

In this chapter, which is really educational rather than experimental, I am covering the two other sources of food besides carbohydrates (that we covered at length in Chapter 2), fat and protein. Understanding some technicalities about the quality, the type, the source and the quantity pertaining to each one can really help you improve your health overall, but also become smarter at losing weight. Every component of your plate works together, as in a ballet, to support your precious body functions optimally.

Let's start with fat. This is a tough chapter, because we will have to overcome a major notion and clarify a brewing tug of war. That's the notion and very strongly anchored belief that "fat makes us fat." Science has evolved, more is known (or finally acknowledged) about calories, the quality of foods, including fats, and the ever growing waist of Americans in a fat-free world. There is a new diet growing in popularity within the rising rate of insulin-resistant population, called the ketogenic diet that even promotes a rather important intake of fat in lieu of carbohydrates, to lose weight.

Fat is also a complicated topic. There has been much controversy lately about bad, versus not so bad fat. The war is between animal based and plant based fats. I hear the question all the time now: "Veronique, is coconut fat good for me?", or "I am not sure, is butter really bad for my arteries?" To make things even more complicated, even within a category, not good is all good. There is a difference, between butter produced by a grass fed, free roaming cow and by an industrially raised, grains and corn versus grass fed one. Even organically grown olive oil, if chemically altered for shelf life extension can lose its health benefits. And all vegetable oils are not created equal either. So whom to trust anymore and what to eat? I will give you as balanced information as possible. Knowing there are some clear answers, and some grey zones.

Then, I will cover the mighty protein. Because women, in my experience, do not eat enough protein and rely too much on carbohydrates. I can prove it. I have witnessed it so many times. Protein is important for your body in general and for weight loss in particular. In this chapter I will help you understand why you need it, what your minimum intake should be and what the best sources are, including for vegetarians who are so easily deficient.

Fat – Why The Bad Rap?

It all boils down to the fact that years ago, we were told - and sold on the fact - that fat-free foods were better for optimal health and weight loss. And fat was bad. It was a very easy way to get rid of extra calories of course. Fat was bad, because:

One gram of fat carries 9 calories versus a gram of carbohydrate or protein which only carry four calories. Also, fat aids cholesterol absorbtion and triggers cardiovascular diseases by clogging your arteries – or so we thought…

Here it was: "cut the fat, and save double the calories". Therefore, the 80's birth and blossoming of a new world of fat free dairy, fat free cookies and sweets, fat- reduced dressings, low-calorie this and low- calorie that. I have met so many fat phobic women in my classes. But it makes sense, psychologically, right? Fat is fat. Fat equals fat in your body. Fat is not a pleasant word.

Besides, we were also told that fat was clogging our arteries and raising our bad cholesterol. Hence the birth of margarine and plant based oils. But now new data and science is showing that good fat can help you reverse cardiovascular diseases and Type 2 diabetes, and prevent dementia, cancer and other diseases. There are studies also questioning the fact that saturated fats even create cardiovascular diseases when taken in moderation. The advice is to eat healthy saturated fats, principally from grass fed animals, but in moderation. It will behave differently in your body than trans fats. The new villain is sugar. Too much sugar in the blood requires insulin to take it out, if not burnt immediately for energy. Insulin is a fat storing hormone that creates fat via the liver – it is called lipogenesis. This fat then roams into your body raising bad cholesterol and triglycerides, and creating fatty livers.

....

Cogni Data: In our 2016 clinical trial, that promoted nutritional increase in unsaturated fat, and carbohydrates elimination (white carbs and sugar), we saw a statistically significant decrease in total cholesterol (-7%), LDL (-6%), and triglycerides (-30%) in the per protocol analyzed participants. We did not observe a change in HDL or A1c.

....

Let's start with the multiple benefits of fat. According to the RDA, it should represent 20 to 30% of your daily intake for a 1,500 to 2,000 calorie a day diet.

Ninety percent should come from unsaturated fat and 10% maximum from saturated fat. Some high fat, low carbohydrate diet recommendations go as high as 60-70% of calories coming from fat and as low as 20g of carbohydrates a day which can cause an issue with vitamins, antioxidants and fiber intake. I am not promoting this and there are special books written about that. This low carb, high fat diet is gaining traction especially within the Type 2 diabetes world and carboholic population. And if it helps, I am all for it. But in this book, we will stick to a rather balanced diet, promoting elimination of white carbs and sugar, increasing non starchy vegetables and good fat (including in nuts).

My fat intake is now 40% (initially at 30%) for a 1,200-1,300 calorie a day regimen. I have started to eat more nuts, creamy sheep and goat yogurts and many avocados. And I am cooking with coconut oil and coconut milk more often, even adding it to my smoothies.

Before we explain the difference between saturated fats, poly and mono-unsaturated fats, and trans fats, which do not all behave equally in your body, let's look at the multiple benefits of good fat in general:

- Helps you absorb vitamins A, D, and E. Without fat in your diet, these vitamins will not deliver any benefits and will go in and out of your body
- Supports your nervous system. Phospholipids and sterol cholesterol, all forms of fat, provide a protective barrier to your cells.
- Lowers LDL and triglycerides
- Nourishes your skin, nails and hair
- Necessary for your brain to function, and you to be happy
- Does not create insulin spikes unless carbohydrates and even protein (when there are not enough carbohydrates)
- Delays sugar absorption therefore insulin spikes (remember Chapter 2)

Cogni-Tip:

Good fat can help you lose weight in an interesting manner. But not all fats are equal.

When combined with carbohydrates, which are usually part of your meal, fat will allow for lower insulin spikes, and therefore less fat storing. In a nutshell, if you eat a sugar free yogurt, you will have a bigger insulin spike than if you had a 2% fat yogurt. And if not burned quickly, remember the chapter on sugar, extra glucose will be stored as fat. Even if the 2% yogurt has overall more calories, the yogurt fat will be burned for energy.

Now, why is good fat helping you lose weight, even if it has double the calories than carbohydrates?

- Fat must be burned when consumed and is not easy to store
- It does not spike your insulin, the fat storing hormone, because it does not impact this hormone
- It makes you and your brain more satisfied, for longer. You will have less cravings, believe me
- Good fat does not trigger inflammation, unlike sugar (or trans fats)
- Fat will not trigger water retention, a phenomenon associated with high carbs, highly inflammatory diets

Cogni-Tip:

Fat can boost your metabolism and help you lose weight. One of the major reason is that unlike sugar/carbohydrates it does not impact insulin, the fat storing hormone.

To summarize, and as demonstrated in more studies now, when you increase your consumption of good fat and lower your consumption of bad carbohydrates, for the same amount of total calories (let's stay grounded in respecting this for the sake of your weight loss efforts), you will lose weight, or even more weight (than on a high carbohydrate diet).

Furthermore (and you will conduct the experiment), when you eat more fat during a meal, you feel more satiated and you will snack less than when you eat more carbohydrate rich meals. As an example a piece of salmon with vegetables versus a plate of spaghetti with meat balls and tomato sauce or a pizza at lunch, will increase your chances to keep cravings away.

Let's look at fats, who is bad, who is good?

This part of the chapter has been very challenging because there is no black or white here. There are a few established facts but there is also recent complications and new science that have fueled a controversy mostly backed by powerful food lobbies. But before we go there let's look at the different types of fat we have. Promised, I will keep it simple.

Saturated versus unsaturated fat, what is the difference?

- **Saturated fat** is usually derived from animals, and is solid at room temperature. We are talking about meat, cheese, milk and dairy in general. Coconut nut oil, is also considered a saturated fat.

- **Unsaturated fat** is mostly derived from plants, but also from fish, and is usually liquid. To make things more complicated, there are different types of unsaturated fats, the **mono and the poly-unsaturated** kinds that have to do with chemical structure.

- The food industry can take any good fat and make it bad, by adding a Hydrogen atom. There are vegetable based oils that the process makes solid. They are called **trans fats**. And why? Because it allows the fat to have a longer shelf life by postponing fat rancidity. It makes the fat able to withstand light, temperature changes etc. These are really the bad fats! Combined with high fructose sugar, in processed foods, it is a deadly combination.

To make things even more complex, saturated fats are not made only of saturated fats. As an example butter is 60% saturated and 40% unsaturated. Coconut fat is 90% saturated and 10% unsaturated.

Let's look at different fats, their benefits or issues, and where we can find them:

Type of Fat: Monounsaturated fats or MUFAs

Benefits/Issues:

- Lowers bad cholesterol or LDL
- Raises good cholesterol or HDL

Attention to palm oil, which is a good fat but has to come from the plant and NOT the kernel. It is replacing trans fats in multiple processed foods. Also there are environmental issues with deforestation due to extreme harvesting. You may check if it is a sustainably obtained oil.

Avoid canola oil, touted as healthy. It is an industrialized oil that has lost its MUFAs due to multiple chemical processes.

Avoid grape seed oil, another highly processed and industrial oil.

Found in: Olive oil, olives, macadamias, almonds, pecans, cashews, peanuts, avocados (and avocado oil), hazelnut, walnut, sesame seeds and nut butters.

Type of Fat: Polyunsaturated fats

mostly Omega 3 and Omega 6 fats

Benefits/Issues:

- Lowers LDL
- Omega 3: brain health, joints, HDL, weight loss
- Omega 6: is also beneficial but can be inflammatory in too big quantities

Important: The healthy ratio Omega 6 to Omega 3 in our food was around 1 to 1. It is the imbalance between Omega 3 and 6 that is the issue and promotes cardiovascular disease and inflammation.

Nowadays it is 15 to 16.7-1.1[1]

1: *The importance of the ratio of omega-6/omega-3 essential fatty acids. Simopoulos AP. .NCBI. Biomed. Pharmacop. 2002 Oct;56(8):365-79*

Omega 3 found in:

- Wild caught oily fish such as salmon, mackerel, and sardines.
- Fish oil supplements.
- Grass fed animals especially beef
- Plants such purslane (a green plant) and hemp, chia and flax seeds are rich in Omega 3.

Omega 6 found in:

- Safflower oil
- Corn oil
- Corn fed meats/poultry

Type of Fat: Saturated fats

Butter, ghee, lard and coconut oil

Benefits/Issues:

Even if coming from pastured raised animals, and butter is making a comeback, I will caution on the quantity! It is still fat!

And it will clog your arteries!

Coconut is also a saturated fat but it behaves differently than other saturated fats. There is a special paragraph later on coconut oil.

Found in: Meat, poultry, cheese, dairy mostly.

Type of Fat: Trans fats

Benefits/Issues:

They appear on labels but there is a caveat. It has only to be labeled if it is has more than 0.5g per serving.

You should not exceed 2g a day or 18 calories for a 2,000 calorie diet.

They trigger inflammation, reduce HDL, and create bad LDL.

Found in: Processed foods including protein bars, snacks and so forth that you may like to have from time to time.

Also used in baking, so beware when you buy these pastries, even at a good baker's shop. Ask what kind of fat they use!

Crisco®, Pam® spray, margarine, coffee creamers contain trans fats.

A word about cooking. I always have that question. What happens when oils and fats are submitted to high temperatures, do they go bad? Yes, they do because they oxidize and become harmful to your health.

- Coconut, avocado, palm, butter, lard, ghee (butter without the sugars and proteins) can withstand high temperatures. When they start to fume, or even worse, get brown, you know you have reached the dangerous oxidization point. The highest point is usually 325 degrees F.

- Olive oil should be kept for mild heat or salads

One word about coconut — friend or foe?

Coconut oil is 90% saturated fat. But half of the saturated fat is made of lauric acid. Lauric acid transforms in your body unlike other saturated fats and becomes a super food. So I vouch for coconut oil but again, it has to be pure and of good quality. Coconut oil can withstand high temperature for cooking, but can leave a little taste not to everybody's liking. I sometimes mix half coconut and olive oil when I cook.

It is delicious also added to smoothies (1 tbsp. is +/- 100 calories) and will provide this satiety factor to the smoothie. Some people now add it in their coffee in the morning for the same reason.

Still find it confusing?

Nowadays, what matters more is the quality of the food you put in your mouth than anything else, beyond the quantity of course. And its purity. Recently I bought nuts at the airport and reading the label I realized they had been "sprayed" with cotton seed oil. Cotton seed oil is not regulated as a food, is cheap and is full of pesticides. It is added to a lot of processed foods as a cheap fat and/or to increase shelf life because it has been chemically altered. So I was shocked to discover than even a pack of nuts could be polluted like this.

There are a lot of fake olive oils, nut butters that are not 100% nuts, false claims or lack of transparency on oils and other fats labels. You have to increase your curiosity factor.

But when it comes to your health and weight loss, do not be afraid of good fats, even good old saturated butter. As long as you watch your total calories! You will perform the experiment in this chapter. You move just 10% of your daily intake from starchy carbohydrates to fat heavy foods such as avocado or a good yogurt (2% is enough) and you will feel better, have less cravings and lose weight. Even for the same number of total calories!

To Summarize:

Eat good mono and poly unsaturated fats and avoid processed and fried foods as much as you can. Don't be too afraid of saturated fats as long as they come from pasture and organically raised animals. But be conscientious that 1g of fat is 9 calories and that it adds up quickly. When deciding to increase fat intake, I highly recommend to watch total calorie intake with an app or keeping a food diary. Nuts and good cheese, extra spoons of olive and coconut oils can build up to an extra 500 to 1,000 calories a day.

Now let's look at our other friend, one very often neglected by women, the protein.

The Mighty Protein

I have noticed so many times that women do not pay enough attention to protein. And often lean on a high carb and sweet diet that completely works against them when it comes to weight loss. So the goal of this section is to insure that you become more aware of how much protein you eat, from what sources and that you pay attention to it, especially if you start to move and exercise more.

Proteins are chains of amino-acids. Each amino acid has specific roles within your body, and not just for growing and repairing your cells and muscles. They provide a long list of benefits to name a few:

- Strengthen your immune system
- Transportation of lipids or fat, minerals and oxygen
- Creation of other proteins with important internal roles at every level of our body
- Balance of fluid electrolytes

Proteins get dismantled in amino acids in the digestive process by specific enzymes and then, can go and do perform all their little miracles.

Cogni-Tip:

There are 9 essential amino-acids out of the 20 available in foods. The body is capable of producing its own amino-acids except for these 9 essential ones that MUST be taken from food sources. Vegetarians must be VERY CAREFUL about what they are eating as many plants lack certain essential amino acids.

Essential	Conditionally Non-Essential	Non-Essential
Histidine	Arginine	Alanine
Isoleucine	Asparagine	Asparatate
Leucine	Glutamine	Cysteine
Methionine	Glycine	Glutamate
Phenylalanine	Proline	
Threonine	Serine	
Tryptophan	Tyrosine	
Valine		
Lysine		

Proteins from animal origin provide all the 20 amino acids. Vegetables, grains and fruits do not provide all amino acids. For example rice is rich in methionine and low in lysine and beans are the reverse. Professional vegetarians/vegans have mastered the art of combining vegetables in order to provide the 9 essential amino acids. New science shows that unlike initially thought, you do not need to eat all same amino acids at the same time. The body can store those it has in excess. So for vegetarian and vegans, the balance has to be looked over days. You do not always have to combine rice and beans.

Vegetarians/vegans find their proteins in protein rich vegetables and carbohydrates such as legumes (beans and lentils), nuts (and now nut milks a, yogurts and cheeses), soy and its multiple preparations such as tofu, tempeh, and if allowed, in eggs and yogurts. Some people will eat fish, but not meat or poultry, some will allow or not animal by-products such as dairy, eggs and cheese as a philosophy or for a pure dietary reason.

But at the end of the day, we all need to eat enough protein and enough of each ones of the essential amino acids.

To go back to the past, one of the reasons diets such as the original Atkins, The Dr. Dukan diet and other high protein diets were so popular is that on the contrary to fat or carbohydrates, amino acids cannot create fat in your body. However again, not everything is black or white. Too much protein in your diet, and not enough carbohydrates, and will get your body in survival mode for energy. A phenomenon called gluconeogenesis will use protein as glucose and it will still spike your insulin. Hence the need for balanced meals.

If you eat a pure diet of protein (fat in meats not included) you will shrink away very fast, but it is not recommended. A high protein diet, not accompanied with extreme physical effort like athletes, has many dangerous side effects, such as kidney problems or even failure, especially as water consumption must be increased with higher protein intake. By-products of protein such as nitrogen and creatinine must be excreted. Also because the pH of your blood will become more acidic on a high protein diet, the body will have to extract extra minerals such as calcium from your bones to rebalance the pH and this can lead to osteoporosis.

Constipation will occur due to lack of fiber if this high protein diet is not accompanied by sufficient fiber-rich vegetables, fruits and nuts intake. High protein diets rich in meats and poultry, especially industrially raised ones can elevate your blood pressure.

Again, the lesson learned here is that everything we do when it comes to food must be done with balance. How many proteins should you eat every day is crucial. Not too many, not too few.

The answer is: it depends. Your physical activity will have an impact on your need to support and replenish your muscle mass and cells structure.

You must have heard about the number of chickens some athletes eat every day to maintain and grow their muscles mass. But we are here with regular ladies like you and me.
In general, the RDA, based on a 1,500 to 2,000 calorie diet a day recommends 25 to 30% of daily calorie intake to come from protein (remember there are proteins everywhere including in nuts, grains, vegetables and fruits). But everybody eats a little bit differently so ratios are not always optimal.

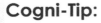

Cogni-Tip:

There is a simple formula that takes into account your weight to help guide your needs. There are other more sophisticated formulas that use lean body mass, but you need a special measurement/scales to find that out. I believe in life you have to keep things simple. Women in general do not need more that 50g a day and men around 70g. However types, body size and level of activity can influence the needs. Use this formula:

$$\frac{\textbf{Your weight in pounds X 0.8}}{\textbf{2.2}}$$

As an example a 170 lb. woman will need 62g a day

If you are more active and do strength and cardio training on a regular basis you need to use this formula:

$$\frac{\textbf{Your weight in pounds X 1}}{\textbf{2.2}}$$

So a 170 lb. woman would need 77g a day in that situation

So what are your protein needs?

Activity Level	Daily Needs of Protein in Grams
Non physically active	
Exercising seriously – at least one hour in a day	

Now you will ask: "what are the best sources for protein?" You will notice there is protein in every food, but mostly in animal based sources. If you are an average woman and you eat three decks of cards of steak in a day you would get approximately the 60g you need. On the other hand you would have to eat 3 to 4 cups of lentils and beans. But these are unbalanced meals. Mixing and matching is crucial as every food will bring different nutrients, besides just proteins and amino-acids.

Protein Content in Food

Source	Protein Content	Other Nutrients
1 oz. meat or poultry	7g in 1oz. or One deck of cards = 3oz. = 21g	Very rich in saturated fats
1 oz. fish	7g	Rich in Omega 3, especially salmon, mackerel, sardines
1 cup vegetarian-based sources	14g in tofu, +/-30g in 1 cup soybeans or tempeh/seitan. Quinoa 8g/cup	No saturated fats
1 cup milk/yogurt or 1 oz. cheese	6-8g	Rich in saturated fats

Source	Protein Content	Other Nutrients
1 Egg	7g	+/-5g of fat in yolk = 50 calories out of 70-80 calories
Nuts and seeds	1 tbs. nut butter = 3-4g, 1/2 oz. nuts = 7g	good fat source
1 cup cooked legumes	18g lentils to 15-18g most other beans	very rich in fiber!
Other vegetables	1 cup cooked vegetables or 2 cups raw vegetables = 3-5g	highest are mostly green/cruciferous such as spinach, cabbage, kale, green collards, etc. Also rich in fiber
Carbohydrates	1 slice whole bread=3g and 1 cup cooked whole rice/pasta=6g	source of fiber and whole carbs

Now, take 5 minutes and calculate how much protein you ate yesterday or today, do a quick math:

Yesterday I ate _____ grams of proteins

_____ % came from animals (meats or by-products such as dairy and eggs)

_____ % came from other foods

As a vegetarian/vegan, or even as a non-vegetarian, you may notice, and I will share the story of Deb later, that you may end up eating too many pizzas, rice and other starchy carbohydrates. The result is either that you do not get enough protein and/or are eating too many starches. Besides, if you are a vegetarian/vegan and are a beginner, you must do your research and learn your best sources. It is an art today as many new protein sources for vegetarians are industrially concocted and loaded with flavor enhancers, thickening agents, texture enhancers and more. Look at mixing and matching vegetables/carbohydrates/nuts for optimal amino-acid combination intake, starchy carbohydrates control and fiber content. Here are a few good resources I found:

www.vegsoc.org, this is the site of The Vegetarian Society
www.vrg.org, this is the site for The Vegetarian Resource Group.

For recipes:

www.vegetarianrecipes.net
www.vegetariannutrition.net

My advice to my growing number of vegetarian/vegan clients is as follows:

- Take the time for a few days to check how much protein you are eating

- Note the sources for your protein intake

- If you are extremely strict – no meat nor fish, and no animal based products (no eggs, no milk, and no cheese), you have to supplement your diet with nuts, nut butters or nut based milks and dairy, or a plant based protein daily shake. Usually a scoop will provide 10 to 20g of protein. There are many wonderful options now. Protein are extracted from plants such as hemp, peas, artichokes, quinoa, some seeds or nuts such as pumpkin, amaranth etc.

Cogni-Tip:

When purchasing a protein powder, no matter the origin, you must check the following:

- The amino-acids content. You must make sure it provides a good balance of the 9 essential amino acids

- The source must be preferably non GMO (difficult to know however), and organic (again difficult to really guarantee)

- "Naturally grown" as a claim does not mean anything

- Soy is one of the highest industrially and GMO raised crop. Furthermore, if you have a history of estrogen dependent cancer in your family, it should be avoided, as soy as a molecule mimics the structure of estrogen

For non-vegetarians, the go to powder is whey. Whey is a by-product of the production of cheese. Proteins are extracted from it. It is still the best when it comes to proteins for muscles protection. However it is also coming from highly industrialized milk. So you do not know the real quality of the powder.

Beware also of all the added plusses, to raise the price, such as enzymes for improved digestion, minerals or probiotics, green foods, and extra fiber. They are nice to have, but they may be redundant with the other supplements you already take. Sugar is contained naturally in plants, and even in milk, but check if anything was added for taste improvement such as either real sugar, or sweeteners especially when the powder is flavored, including vanilla and chocolate. I buy my powders with no added flavors.

A new trend is to buy collagen protein powder. It is very rich in minerals and is extracted from bones and marrows, but again, you do not know from what cows or animals it may be coming from. I personally like this powder from time to time as the collagen is a form of protein, created by the body that acts like a glue for your tissues and bones. To give you an idea, synthetic collagen is used as an injection for cosmetic surgery. As we age, collagen levels go down, hence tissue sagging. I am always leery of marketing claims, a home-made bone broth will also provide you what you need, but the collagen powder is a nice change.

A note of caution. I am not a big fan of protein powders, nor of protein bars. I prefer to eat natural food in their God given initial state. However, again, if you have a hard time getting your daily protein needs, or are really on the go a lot, a good protein source based powder or bar will be a great surrogate. Better than a muffin anyhow. But please do not make this your routine. The maximum I will allow my clients to substitute a meal for a powder, because of their complicated lifestyle is one protein powder smoothie a day. I am even a lesser fan of bars. Carry varied nuts instead and check your bar labels, especially the ingredients.

Protein bars check list:

- Source of the proteins – you will not get a breakdown of amino acids, unlike powders

- Added fats. Is there any trans fats, or saturated fats? It is OK in small quantities, but what if you eat a bar every day?

- Added fiber, if any. What is the source?

- Check the amount of carbohydrates. Besides the fiber, it is all sugar at the end! So a bar with 25g of carbohydrates — minus 5 g of fiber — is almost 20g of pure sugar! Or 4 teaspoons, do you really need that?

- Additives. If it's not comprehensible, it's not necessary.

I know a fitness trainer who lives on protein bars. She does not eat a lot. She exercises a lot. She cannot lose weight. She is 20 pounds overweight. She has a bar for breakfast and one for lunch! Yes, she has enough protein but she is not nourishing her body. Protein bars are full of chemical ingredients and sugars. She has created inflammation in her body and is vegetables and fiber depleted. This is why she can't lose the weight. She is eating chemicals.

I recommend to vary your protein powders as well if you take one frequently. I use a plant based one, a collagen one and sometimes I also take whey powder. I personally take a protein powder shake when I know I skipped, will skip a meal, and especially on days when I run or go to the gym.

To Summarize

The protein story is easier than the fat story. Eat your 50-60g a day minimum from varied sources of animal and plant based sources. Do not go crazy on protein either, you do not need them if you are not a professional athlete and you may end up creating insulin spikes if you eat too much protein and not enough carbohydrates. Use powders and especially bars uniquely when in a rut, on the go a lot, or initially, especially as a vegetarian, very protein deprived. And check your labels. My solution for extra protein is nuts or a yogurt, which are natural sources. I avoid cheeses, very high in saturated fats.

I hope you have enough information now to eat your good fat without fear and enough protein for weight loss. Let's enjoy a few experiments to boost your nutrition IQ and confidence level.

Deb's story and amazing weight loss journey

Deb is a beautiful person, inside and out. A gentle soul. She came into our clinical trial, frustrated at not being able to lose weight at 58. Deb was a true vegetarian with serious carbohydrates and sugar addictions. She was the pizza, rice and pasta lover, experiencing day long cravings triggered by this highly starchy carbohydrate regimen. Vegetables were not really on her menu. Cooking wasn't' either.

The CogniDiet® was a revelation for her. She did not know carbohydrates turned into glucose in her blood. She said learning that was her biggest aha of the program. She then learned the difference between fast and slow release, whole and white, starchy or fiber rich carbohydrates. For her, a carbohydrate was a carbohydrate. She also realized she was seriously protein-underfed and relied on take away, frozen meals and restaurants to get her meals.

She knew this was a not very convenient way of living. She was also fat phobic, like most of women I work with, and as a consequence was constantly spiking her glucose blood sugar level, triggering insulin release, and storing fat a little bit more every day.

She was pre-diabetic with a hemoglobin A1c level of 6.0 at the beginning of the trial and she finished still at 6.0. The threshold for pre-diabetes type 2 is a hemoglobin A1c of 5.7. She called me in June 2017 to tell me her hemoglobin A1c was at 5.5. So it took another 6 months after the trial, to lower the average sugar level in her blood and by the way to lose another 16 pounds.

When she joined the trial, she did not know where to start to lose weight. She knew she had to change her diet and her lifestyle. She was thirsty for information. She felt very crappy, her words. Constantly tired and somewhat depressed. She understood very quickly in the clinical trial that she would have to learn to cook for herself.

She was very frustrated about her constant sugar cravings and felt guilty about it, blaming her own lack of willpower. She was one of these very quiet, yet focused and disciplined participants. You know, there is always the constant questioner, the bigger than life, and the know - it - all participant in every group. But Deb had this aura of calmness, maybe because she is a teacher.

The first action Deb took was to eliminate the white carbs and the sugar. She went with an axe. This is how she dealt with her cravings:

1. She mentally pictured what she liked but would not eat anymore and created a secret list. She told herself she would postpone eating them until the end of the trial. By the way, she never went back to these sugary treats at the end of the trial and continued to lose weight.

2. She also took a tough approach to her journey. She decided enough was enough. She toughened up and eliminated all sugary and processed foods overnight. She went cold turkey.

She also started to experiment with protein powder as a supplement and added eggs and yogurt and cottage cheese to her meals to supplement on protein. She was initially getting too much of her protein from legumes, including beans, which are still quite high in carbohydrates. She used her transformation journey by turning her creativity into cooking with carb substitutes.

She replaced white flour pizza crust with cauliflower crust. She bought a spiralizer and cooked zucchini noodles. She made it a game to discover new vegetables every week. We shared many recipes. When I interviewed her for this book in July 2017 she told me she was now making her own almond milk, chia pudding, and had acquired the best cooking accessories to feed, no pun intended, her new passion for cooking.

She lost 23 pounds in 12 weeks, and when I saw her for the 6 months follow up she had lost another 16 pounds as you heard earlier. She was more proud about the 16 pounds, that she did on her own, than anything else. She told me she did not even realize how because "I am eating naturally, I cook for myself, I am rather disciplined, but I am not really paying attention to calories, nor portions". And I answered: "your body feels the love, you are nourishing it. You are optimizing all its functions. You are getting rid of chronic inflammation"

Here are a few of her quotes:

"I am not feeling deprived. I have no cravings. I don't want sugar anymore. I have lost the taste for it. I am now content with a piece of 85% chocolate once in a while"

"I feel like a big burden has been taken away from my shoulders. A feeling of helplessness. A sense I could never win this war with sugar. Little did I know how badly I was eating. It was so simple to change."

"I really started to feel a difference when I became more disciplined with my proteins. I never knew I was so deprived. When we did the protein count, and did a diary for a few days, I found out some days I was eating a mere 30g and I am a tall girl."

"At 58 I feel like I have a new life, a new perspective, a new confidence. And come to think about it, I owe it to cauliflower and coconut oil, LOL!"

"I have realized it is not that hard to get in control. You just have to decide it is about you. You use sabotaging thoughts to allow you to continue to have the wrong behaviors. You decide this person will be upset if you don't eat her cake. Not true. Just say no gently, and it is OK."

"I never realized it was so fulfilling and joyful to cook healthy foods. And not that complicated. Keep it simple, play with spices and a few ingredients."

Deb went through and entire pantry and cooking revolution and has become an active recipe sharer with our group.

From flour based crusts	to cauliflower or almond flour based crusts
From pasta	to zucchini or squash based noodles
From plant based protein	to more eggs, protein powder (plant based), dairy
From low-fat everything	to full fat dairy, low sugar/high fat chocolate
From frozen and fast food	to home cooked meals, rich in vegetables
From Pam®	to good olive oil and coconut oil

Be inspired my friends. Deb does not feel that cooking or food shopping has taken anything away from her social or personal life. The rewards in increased energy, self-confidence and well-being largely outweigh the extra hour a day she spends in the kitchen or shopping.

She told me some of her friends don't understand how she does it. When they ask her how she lost almost 48 pounds, she has no real secret diet, or supplement or any medication. She tells them she just eats fresh. She mentioned there is a lot of work to do to make people understand that bread and rice and all these carbs become sugar in your blood. There is a lot of unfortunate ignorance still that prevents people with the best intentions to really succeed at losing weight. But I also feel confident this book will help you lose weight naturally and increase your overall nutrition IQ.

Now enjoy your experiments!

· ·

This Week's Experiments

Experiment #1: Know your fat intake – and vary them

Calculate the fat intake you want to achieve within your overall calorie intake. Let's say that for 1,200 calories, you want 33% or 400 calories coming from fat, or approximately to simplify 45g. Us a calorie counter app.

Where are these 45g coming from? Observe your diet over 3 days. Is it coming mostly from meat and animal based fats, therefore mostly saturated? What type of poultry or meat are you eating? Is it grass fed, organic, natural (which means nothing), are you on a budget and buying the most economical sources?

Or do you eat fish too? Be careful nowadays not to eat fish more than twice a week as it contains too much mercury, chemicals and even plastic! Avoid farm-raised fish too. Are you eating a lot of dairy, or are you adding coconut oil in everything?

I always advertise a balanced diet with multiple sources of fat. Remember that our U.S. Omega3/Omega 6 balance is out of whack. Experiment with chia or flaxseeds in your diet, add a fish oil supplement or fatty fish, and make sure you get to a 4/1 Omega 3/Omega 6 ratio to combat inflammation.

I am not asking you to become obsessive about it, but you have to check how you are eating and understand what you put in your body before you can change. You may realize all this packaged/processed food brings you more than 20% of trans fats. That my friend is not good for your health, but is also sabotaging your weight loss efforts.

Experiment #2: Know your protein intake — and vary them

Please calculate your minimal protein intake and then check how much of it you eat, and what are the sources. Write this in your daily food diary. Do a few days, so that you can see variations.

$$\frac{\text{Your weight in pounds X 0.8}}{2.2}$$

If you are more active and do strength and cardio training on a regular basis you need to use this formula:

$$\frac{\text{Your weight in pounds X 1}}{2.2}$$

What have you realized? Now, write down your favorite foods with high protein content and get your plan in place. Think about varying your protein sources in multiple ways. Do not always eat steak, fish, or chicken, add soy one day like tofu, or add some egg whites to your omelet in the morning. Have legumes, they are protein and fiber rich. Have a protein rich smoothie in the morning. One scoop of protein powder can give you up to 20g of protein. This experiment is very important for vegetarians/vegans!

It is also important to split your daily protein intake all over the meals and snacks and not just in one meal. Your body wants balance. Try to avoid to have a large amount of protein at one meal, and then none at the next. So make sure there is a protein source at each meal and remember that when you eat carbohydrates, you need to combine them with a protein and a fat.

Experiment #3: Learn to tame your cravings with good fat!

That may seem like a strange experiment to you. But I want you to feel the power of good fat. Do it at breakfast or lunch, when you can observe the impact of the extra fat on your hunger level or cravings in the morning or afternoon.

- Add a half avocado to your lunch for instance, and/or add a high fat yogurt for dessert

- Snack on nuts one day (150 calories around 10 a.m. and another 150 calories around 4 p.m.), and see how it impacts your hunger for lunch and dinner. Warning: nuts are high in calories, so stay in control! 150 calories is approximately 20 to 15 nuts.

- Have a creamy smoothie in the morning for breakfast, including:
   - 15-20g protein powder
   - Vegetables (3/4) and fruits (1/4)
   - Add a half avocado or a good table spoon of coconut fat or mix your smoothie with real coconut milk as your liquid

- Eat a high fat meal with good fat sources (oily fish, full fat dairy, Omega 3 rich seeds, nuts, extra olive oil). I am not saying, go into a fat binge, but be more daring than usual

Questions for the day:

- How are the cravings after the meal, and how long do you stay satisfied?
- How is your hunger level?
- How is your energy level and ability to stay focused?
- How is your appetite at the next meal?
- Have you thought about mid-day snacks as much as usual?

For the fat phobic, once you try this experiment, continue for one week to build your confidence level that good fat does not make you fat.

Just increase your fat intake, while cutting carbohydrates (except vegetables). If you find out you have been more like a 20% fat intake type of person (for overall daily intake in terms of calories) because you are fat phobic, increase to 30% for one week by adding oily fish such as salmon (I know it is expensive, sardines in a can are good and cheaper options), avocados, olive oil, coconut fat in your smoothies etc. At the same time, cut your starchy carbs.

Of course watch your calories, but I am curious to see how your scales will behave. I bet you will have lost weight.

Experiment #4: Know your labels – discover trans fats

Next time you buy any processed foods, a protein bar, or a protein powder, read the label carefully. Discover if there are trans-fat, what kind of oil is used (is it palm oil, cottonseed oil?).

Notice than even in some "good food", the natural product has been adulterated, or replaced with cheaper ingredients:

- Palm oil added to nut butters – Is it palm oil or palm kernel oil?
- Even for packets of nuts, check the ingredients list. I have been more than once surprised that the nuts were protected by cotton seed oil to prevent rancidity.
- "No trans fats claims". Because if it is under 0.5 g per serving, it does not have to be on the label. But even with that claim, look at the ingredients list, you may find some questionable fat sources. And how many servings will you end up eating anyhow?
- Protein bars are a melting pot of ingredients. The sources of fat can be pretty unclear.

Does the label indicate if the oil used is in its natural state? What is the shelf life of that package you are considering buying? Become very curious.

Experiment #5: What has been added to your protein bar or protein powder

Very often, I have this question: "What is a good protein bar or powder?" The challenge as you heard before is that there are a lot of "STUFF" added to any product either for taste, marketing appeal, cost or shelf life issues.

- Soy protein or other protein sources added to nut butters or protein bars

- Is there a sweetener added? Find out which one, is it a form of sugar or an artificial sweetener (I put stevia in that category).

- If it's vanilla, strawberry or chocolate flavored, where is this flavor coming from?

- Are the amino acids well balanced in a vegan protein powder? Do you have the 9 essential ones?

- Compare the claims on the front with the reality of the label and the ingredients

- What is the source of the proteins? If it is whey, does it come from pasture raised cows? In what country? And where? It is not easy to find out but it is worth some research. Same is true when the protein is collagen based, which is rather trendy now with the occurrence of bone broths. But again, who are these cows? How were they fed?

CogniDiet® Book Club Discussion Guide

This week is all about being a label sleuth and yes, also becoming more questioning and aware of what types of fat and protein you put in your body. Maybe you were just buying any protein powder or grabbing any bar at the gym' store? Are you eating enough proteins? Have you realized you are still eating too many carbohydrates, and you feel stuck?

This week is for all of you to bring some protein powders, protein or snack bars and some labels and just play with them at the discussion group.

- **Compare a few products labels, protein bars or powders that you use**

- **Have you discovered you are not eating enough or too much protein? How could you increase this level with varied sources?**

- **How was your morning smoothie experiment? Hunger level? Satiety? Cravings?**

- **Are you even eating enough fat? It is usually recommend to have at least 20% of your calorie requirement in fat, preferably not trans fats**

- **Were you inspired by Deb's transformation? What do you think of her story?**

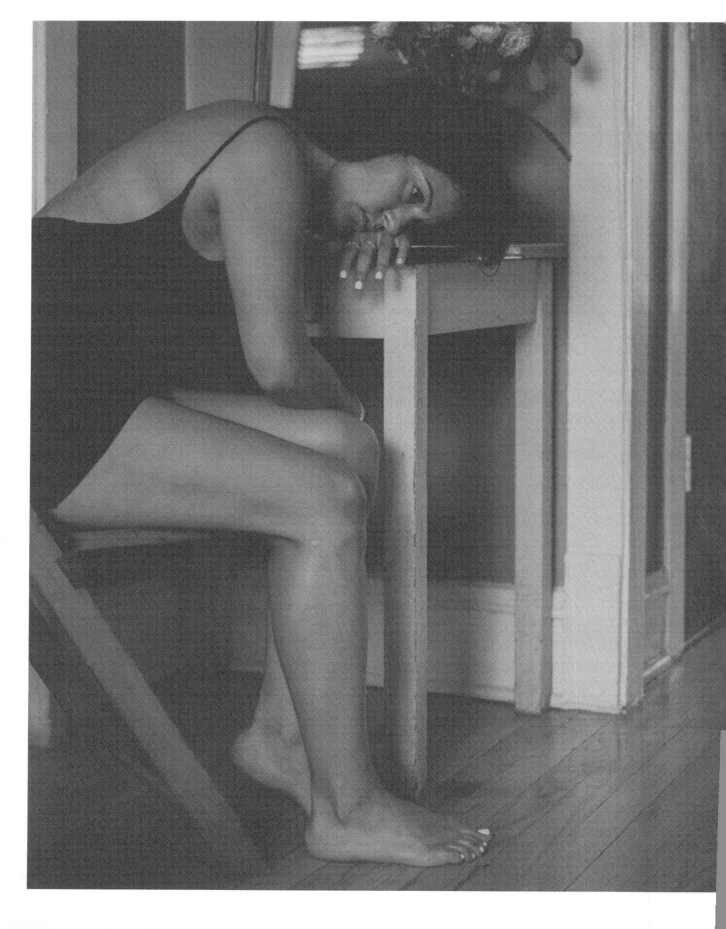

Chapter 9

I Don't Let Emotions Guide My Mouth!

Besides stress, a great saboteur of good intentions, emotions at large can get in the way of your weight loss efforts. In a BIG way. And we have not really covered this yet. This book is not a psychotherapy book, but at least we can help you get in the saddle and start making some changes. Our plan is to help you detect - to start with - and then approach emotions with a novel eye and attitude before we dive into the pretzels bag after a big ugly fight!

Emotions are very diverse, not always known to the person experiencing them. And we all react differently to similar situations. We come with our own baggage, expectations and pre-conceived notions. I can see scorn here, when you could only see irony. One of my nemesis has been the emotion known as frustration, especially when things are not going my way. A contrariety, a setback, an obstacle and boom, here was the chocolate. It took me a while to understand that what was behind the frustration was a feeling that I had no control on a situation or event. My deeper emotion was the need to be in control. Yes, I am a little bit of a control freak. So I had to learn to put things into perspective and let go. It was in fact very freeing, it got my cortisol level down and most of my cravings tamed. And yes I used a few techniques I will share with you in this chapter.

I have witnessed successful participants, doing very well for weeks or months with their diet, and all of a sudden getting off track. It is usually linked to an unplanned event or situation. And again, it may have been stress related, or just fatigue. Stress is not an emotion, it is a situation. But stress is always associated with underlying emotions. I therefore started an emotional eating class in the spring of 2017, and I want to give a little practical flavor of what you can do to help yourself in these situations.

Cogni-Tip:

We literally stuff ourselves often to get the pain away, to avoid an uncomfortable truth, to fill a void, to chase away a feeling that does not make our brain happy. Reflect on this very important statement.

Think about the number of times you may have numbed your emotion with a snack! I remember one day having a difficult discussion with my boss. He was telling me some not so good news about a job transfer. It was not bad news, but I was not happy about the move. I became emotional, not professional, I must admit. Not crying, but showing I felt it was not fair. I was very unhappy about this transfer, at least initially. He stayed professional but I could see he did not know what to do with me. He mumbled a few insipid on-script clichés. All of a sudden however, he opened his desk drawer and started to eat some liquorish candies out of a bag, even offering some to me. In hindsight, he was suppressing his emotions. I knew he liked me and did not know what to say, how to compose himself in front of my disappointment. He must have felt guilty and personally moved by my disappointment. True story.

This week, I am going to ask you to find out your dominant emotions, positive or negative. They may be different at home or at work, or in different situations or people around you. Oh yes, my mother, whom I adore, knows my push buttons! The list of emotions here below is not exhaustive. I will ask you to find out which ones are the most common and the strongest. Some people tell me their eating is not associated with emotions and in this case you may choose to skip this chapter, or you may decide to stay with me and learn a thing or two.

Select your emotions based on their occurrence and their link to food as a response. Then after careful thinking, rank your top 3 or 5:

Your Emotions Examples:	Situations/Persons Associated with the Emotion. *Do you notice a pattern?*	Rank them
Joy		
Anger		
Fear		
Jealousy		
Happiness		
Anxiety		
Frustration		
Loneliness		
Enthusiasm		
Depression		
Other emotions you may experience:		

When we conduct this experiment in our classes, I have noticed that some participants struggle with even detecting and understanding their basic emotions. There is no thinking straight after the fact when going to get the latte with a cookie. Some emotions may be quite uncomfortable and personal as we said earlier. It's imperative that you try to find out, and face, your biggest sabotaging emotions. But they may be deeply hidden, repressed, extremely hurtful, stemming from childhood or a life trauma. In this case, my sincere advice is to speak to a psychotherapist and understand with their help what the roots of these problems are. This is beyond the realm of my abilities.

The goal of this chapter is to give you practical tools to at least deal with these emotions for the short term and start to think and take actions for the longer term - if you decide to deal with them once and for all.

Two "Non" Emotions: Boredom and Stress

Before we start however I want to clarify a point. There are two "non "emotions that I hear about all the time. They are not emotions. They may trigger cravings, but they are not emotions:

1. Boredom! Boredom is a sense of vacuum and emptiness because your mind is not busy. We live in a world over-crowded with empty activities and noise that in truth are not always productive or conducive to happiness. You may sit at home, in the TV room after a long day. You finished checking your Facebook, emails, special sales on Ebay® or your perfect mate on Match.com (somebody told me this matching activity was creating a lot of stress in her life!). You are not preparing dinner before one hour and switch on the TV. You watch it mindlessly. You are bored. You go to the fridge and open it to find something to get you "busy". Chewing, munching, sucking, foods or drinking is an activity. You just can't stay still. However, do not confuse boredom with loneliness.

INSTANT Cogni-Shift:

Next time boredom happens to you, take a few seconds, breathe deeply as you learned, and examine the situation. Measure your hunger level. And if you feel bored, cherish this moment of calm and precious time alone. Read a book or a magazine, do a mini-meditation, or feel gratitude. But boredom is not an emotion.

2. The second one is the omnipresent stress. Stress, as we know from Chapter 5, is a very powerful culprit for carbohydrates cravings. Stress can be triggered by multiple situations and present at different levels of intensity (remember a little bit of stress versus stress all the time). You have to go to the root cause of stress and find out if emotions are associated with these top life stressors. In surveys, the following events (not in order of importance) have been highlighted by participants as situations causing the most levels of stress:

    - Death of a loved one
    - Divorce
    - Loss of a job
    - Financial obligations strain
    - Getting married! And this is a happy one.
    - Moving to a new home. Usually, another good one!
    - Chronic illness, accident, injury
    - Emotional problems (depression, anxiety etc.). This one is tricky because stress can trigger serious breakdowns and health issues as you know, then the new health situation creates even more stress. So it is a vicious circle.

To go back to your daily life, we don't expect that you divorce or move every year, unless you are a Hollywood star maybe. But you may experience little bursts of stress, coming and going, and some of them can even be positive. People tell me they are stressed around the year-end holiday, or before a vacation. These are moments when there is too much to do and to plan for at once. We are in a society that tries to do TOO MUCH. Warren Buffet, when interviewed about what where the traits of the happiest people (no, not the richest people), said "it is people who say

NO most of the time". And they are the happiest because they stay in control of their lives.

A divorce on the other hand is a huge stressor and can trigger multiple emotions. It is the emotion created by the divorce that may trigger the need for comfort via food, not the divorce in itself.

Cogni-Tip:

If you feel cravings coming from stress, and there is an underlying emotion(s), please take the time to identify it (them). Is it:

- **Feeling of inadequacy or even failure**
- **Not being in control**
- **Life being taken over**
- **Feeling of losing your identity**
- **Unhappiness**
- **What is your emotion(s)?**

Once you identify the underlying emotion, write it down. It may not be an emotion after all. It may just be that you took on too much to carry on at once! If so, let go of a few things. Prioritize.

Now, Let's Peel the Layers of Your Emotions

Now that you have a better idea about your most important and sabotaging emotions, we are going to start to peel the layers. The emotion must be spelled out, or decomposed into multiple layers. Emotions are complex. But if you look at them with a cold and pragmatic, almost clinical manner, you will be able to, instead on dwelling on the emotion, find your WANTS, and then address them with solutions. This exercise is just to take the drama out of the emotion.

There is another easy way to get over it. Stay focused on your progress and goals, count to five or 10 next time and say to yourself: "It will pass, it will not be resolved with foods, I am stronger than my emotion". This is one of the experiments in this chapter. But if you are not ready for this, here is your homework this week. Identify your emotions and start to peel the layers in understanding why and how it triggers cravings. Use this diary template to note them down.

Day	Meal/Snack	Eating Pattern	Mood/Emotion	How did I eat this? Did I appreciate it?
Monday	Breakfast Egg, toast and coffee	Natural: Ready to go to work, usual, balanced breakfast	No emotions, just a little bit stressed because of traffic	Quickly, no time to savor. I ate at the kitchen bar, not seated
Monday	Snack at 10 a.m. Two muffins with chocolate frosting	Stressed: dealine due at 12 p.m. and not ready for my meeting	Not hungry, Grabbed first thing I saw. Heart beating fast, anxiety high	Stuffed it into my mouth while walking, took one more to my office. I feel bad and guilty

It is important to do this even if you feel there is no emotions, so that you identify your normal eating patterns. Try to do this for a few days.

Once this is done, we will go to the next step, which helps you transform your emotions into actionable solutions. So that the emotion is not fulfilled with food anymore.

I remember this story about a client who had a very difficult relationship with her husband. There were some career related and financial issues, while also coping with a child who needed special care and attention. Let's call her Molly. I feel like sharing her story now and not at the end of the chapter.

Molly's Story: Eating Your Emotions

She had a miserable life and not only had to be major contributor to the family financial situation by having a job but she also had the extra burden to raise the child almost on her own. The child was also going to a special education school which required high parents' involvement. She was a closet eater. With a predilection for EVERYTHING. Sweets, chocolate, ice cream, cakes, chips, you name it.

When she came home, she had no time to cook, and had to do homework with her child. The dinner was usually take-out of some prepared foods. Molly was 50 pounds overweight at 45 and felt ugly, unloved, unfulfilled, over stressed and a total failure as a woman. She was eating too many processed foods and was gulping her unhappiness down with diet soda and hidden snacks. Her child was 8, and she had gained these 50 pounds since his/her birth. She used to be a rather healthy and muscular woman with beautiful green eyes and lustrous chestnut hair.

Her "emotional survival" foods were planted everywhere in her house, car, office. She had chocolate bars in her bra drawer, cookies behind the rice bags on the kitchen shelf. At the office she was hiding her candies, specifically M&Ms® — small and easy to eat almost secretly — in a bag of empty chips! She confessed to me, ashamed and giggling at her own creativity at the same time, that she was a master at even chewing discreetly, almost like a ventriloquist. Nobody really ever saw her munching.

Her mother helped her occasionally but while doing it, was always very critical of everything. The house was a mess, the food was not healthy enough, the child was not taken care of in the best way. She, Molly, looked terrible and unkempt (her mother's words).

The negative emotions were running deep, in spite of the fact that Molly was a Wharton school MBA and had a pretty important job, used to be a very competitive athlete and was doing a phenomenal job with her child. The husband was not emotionally available, escaping the house and his responsibilities most of the time, with busy late night work, weekend business meetings. Well, you know what I am talking about.

She came to me, referred by a friend, who told her she needed to start to put herself first. She knew she ate badly, was over stressed and did not take care of herself. She was at breaking point. She cried a lot during our sessions. She felt so guilty. So instead of talking of salads and healthy snacks, we started to look at peeling the layers of her emotions, and finding out practical solutions, so that she could start to take better care of herself. Emotions were mostly about self-esteem and not feeling good enough because of the constant criticism, or lack of support, of her family. She also felt she had no self-control, when it came to food. And because of that, she felt weak. And because she felt weak, she ate more.

First she started to write down all the things she did RIGHT. She was amazed at how much she was able to put on that list. She was responsible, a taking charge type of person, a caring individual with principles, a wonderful and devoted mother, a successful professional, the family glue, able to multitask and so on. She even managed to describe a few things she liked about her physical appearance.

Then we looked at what was not being taken care of about herself. Here came health, physical energy, me time, exercise, sharing the burden! When she started that list she had her aha moment: she was not asking for help. She was not putting her stake in the ground. We did some pretty insightful comparisons between her behaviors at the office versus at home. At the office, she was all leadership, bossy, competent, respected and assertive. At home, she became timid. So we created a list of things her husband, or mother, could or should take care of instead of her and she sat down with both of them to explain HER NEEDS, once and for all. Here are her words:

- I need appreciation for what I do. A thank you from time to time would not hurt

- I need support and as of next week will go to the gym 3 times a week, so my dear husband, you will have to take care of the child these days, either in the morning or evening

- I will not be in charge of shopping/cooking/nor ordering food twice a week

- I need my mother to help me and not judge me every 5 seconds, so this will have to change. Mom, please support me as usual, thank you, but stop the judging (her mother was floored)

- Every month, I will have a girls night out

- I have invested into a cooking class for couples. Dear husband, we will start to prepare and eat healthier meals TOGETHER

- I am not perfect, but I am bloody well capable and smart and I have been carrying an unrealistic proportion of family responsibilities (she had created a list and it was apparent the husband was performing at best 30%). Men need facts!

- Now I am putting my health back in the family budget as a valuable currency and I will, darn it, make it a priority!

The couple enrolled in a couple therapy program. She also hired a special mentor/baby sitter two nights a week and slowly but surely got the child to accept to have someone else to do his/her homework. This story illustrates how we transformed her emotions, into practical and actionable "wants" and then turned them into an action list.

Cogni-Tip:

Turn your emotions into action steps. Molly went from emotionally draining, internalized and silent self-sabotaging behaviors to empowering and action oriented pragmatic new behaviors. She implemented all the actions she outlined above. She also created a powerful vision board for herself that inspired her every day.

Molly lost 30 pounds over 8 months in 2015! On her vision board she had glued the words "ME FIRST" in big black letters, in the center.

Her husband is still emotionally detached, but has taken on more responsibilities with the child, including at school, and with shopping and cooking. She talked to her mother about her need to stop this constant criticizing and nagging, and the mother made some changes. It is not easy every day. Is it easier most of the days. Molly became so busy with her new plans that she literally forgot to snack. Her own quote in one of our session: "I do not have the time to think about snacks anymore! My life is full of positive experiences and moments. Even my child feels the energy shift". Molly has also made new friends at the gym, on a like-minded health mission, and enjoys the fact she has recovered some of her youth athletic shape and strength. Is her life perfect? No. Is her life better? Yes. Are all the emotions gone? No. Is she dealing better with them? Yes.

Translate Emotions into Wants and Actions

Now I am going to ask you to translate your emotions into wants and then transform your needs into action steps. This is exactly what Molly did. Below I have summarized how you can peel off the subtle layers of your next triggering situation:

Deal With a Triggering Situation

Situation: (Example)

I am very stressed. I have a deadline and I am afraid I will not deliver on time. I must confess that I am not very good at planning or maybe I took on too much!

Emotions and Feeling:	Wants:
Stress, fear and panic	Organizational skills, confidence, calming methods

Food Choices and Eating Patterns:

I am eating a big bag of popcorn and added some chocolates. In fact, eating these foods helps me to procrastinate. I am not hungry. Must be stress.

Short Term Solutions:	Longer Term Solutions:
1. Take a few mental breaks and/or take a snack that will help you focus — a combo of fat/protein/good carbs 2. Set up time bound milestones 3. Ask for a delay perhaps — it will not kill you to ask!	1. Assess your ability to work under tight deadlines 2. Maybe enroll in a special course for better planning skills and project management

Start your own diary, once you have identified your top emotions and tough situations and focus on short and long term solutions. Use the template on the next page.

You will notice, over time, that when you take your life by the reins, and get yourself in a controlling position, solutions may come to you more naturally. You stop the complaining, the self-pity, and the discouragement cycle as you start to see results occur.

Deal With a Triggering Situation

Situation:

Emotions and Feeling:

Wants:

Food Choices and Eating Patterns:

Short Term Solutions:

Longer Term Solutions:

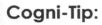

Cogni-Tip:

You do not have to change your life, at every level, overnight! Don't let yourself be overwhelmed by this chapter. Take one challenge at a time. Sit down with a friend, or call me, and prioritize. If the number one issue is mostly eating in your car after a stressful day, take care of that issue first. If it is the sugar craving after each family fight, even a small one, peel away the layers of the issues at hand, and allow a process "à la Molly".

Every change, every improvement, every pound, every one hour exercise slot, every healthy meal, every moment when you become more self-aware and in charge of yourself is A VICTORY. It is a very empowering moments when a client sees a solution versus an obstacle ahead of her.

To help you in your quest, without getting you too self-absorbed, we have designed a few experiments, besides the ones you have to perform in this chapter. Their goals is to dig into your strengths and unearth all the positives in your life, rather that everything that you feel could be better. This helps rewire your brain by focusing on positive pathways that gets all these nice little neuro-transmitters fire with gusto and joy. Some of these experiments will also help you become more assertive with your own priorities, desires and needs.

....

This Week's Experiments

Experiment #1: All the things I love about myself

Take a piece of paper and write all the things you love about yourself. Please don't be shy or timid. If you feel you are not able to write that list, and I have seen this in group meetings, call a few good friends, get them to help you.

It must have to include every aspect of your persona. And not the usual stuff I get from women, in our workshops. Too many times, what comes first, I have noticed, is very often oriented towards caring traits such as compassion, being a good friend or mother, or a great care giver. NO, I also want the hot stuff: "I have a nice nose, I have voluptuous breasts, I am an amazing runner, I am funny, I am a super leader, I am very smart". Cover your intellect, your artistic gifts and talents, your physical features, your heart qualities and your overall personality. And YES, it is also OK to say that you are a tough but fair business woman, or you are a no non sense person, a kick ass competitive spirited cyclist! Start all features with the word I LOVE. I love my blue eyes, my laugh, my humor, my cooking creativity etc. Be bold, be generous with yourself. My wish is for your list to be very long!

I LOVE:

Experiment #2: How can I leverage all these assets for my own benefit?

This one is a continuation of experiment #1. Once you have found out everything you love about yourself, find a way to leverage it for weight loss or even for your life's overall success. As an example, if you love your legs, are you hiding them, are you shy about them? Are you not going to treat them as an asset? Are they muscular and lean because you were gifted by your genes and/or because you are also a pretty good runner? Flaunt them, be proud of them, and love them even more!

Start to wear dresses and skirts to showcase these beautiful legs. You will get compliments. The compliments will boost your self- esteem. You will start to look at other parts of your body and think about how you can flaunt them as well in the future. Maybe the next level is to build a 6 packs!

When you focus on your positive features, your brain lights up and opens doors to many good surprises. You have good feeling thoughts, they travel in the universe and bring you back even more positive treasures. They make you happy and a happy brain may not be so much tempted by sweets after all.

OK, maybe I am exaggerating with the legs, or the hair or the eyes. It's my job to push you out of your shell. Be daring, be adventurous, be innovative. Maybe it's time for a new hairdo, or a new eye makeup style to get them even more beautiful. And if you are more body modest, or not as vain as me, why not focus on your intellectual and personality traits?

- You are a very able organizer at the office. But a disaster when it comes to planning your meals. Please, transfer this skill into your personal life!

- You are a very good and caring friend, and you have many. They like your company. Find one or two who will support YOU in your new health quest by going with you to the gym, or walking once a week together etc.

- You are an amazing cook, but not the healthiest. Well, embark on a new mission to "healthify" all your favorite dishes

- You are very good with managing your family budget. Reflect on the discipline and attention you have while accomplishing this. Why couldn't you transfer this skill to your weekly calorie budget?

You are moving your positive energy into a new endeavor that gets you creative, stretches your limits and pushes you to change. You can start with a small step. A client of mine really loved to bake and also eat what she cooked. She knew it had to stop and she was very sad about it. I also had told her she could not turn to plant based and sugar substitute low calorie recipes because this would continue to encourage her to eat "sugary things". So instead she learned to become creative with vegetables, not just with the recipes, but making a tomato tart look like a piece of art for instance. She continued to use her molds and crafts but became a veggie cooking artsy guru.

So find something to focus your positive energy towards your new life style! Just one thing to start, promised? And every morning when you leave the house, smile at yourself in the mirror and give yourself a compliment.

Experiment #3: Eating after an emotional moment!

This one is a tough one. Because I will ask you to do exactly the reverse of everything I teach you. Next time you have an emotional moment, go to some comfort food, your favorite ones, or anything else that is available. You know in these moments, you are capable to go back in the trash can where you had thrown all these candy bars away or scavenge the office fridge! It is that bad, right? I am not asking you to do this after a very tough and traumatic moment of course. Choose a mild emotion like a small fight, a mild anxiety about going to a party with strangers because you are shy. It could even be a joyful emotion.

You are going for whatever food you can find. Maybe it is still stashed – should not after 9 weeks on the program – in your desk or a secret drawer in your kitchen. This is called the survival stash. Please if you can, observe yourself as you eat. Try to become the observer of the event. What would you write about yourself if you were looking at yourself at that moment?

- How savagely do you unwrap this chocolate bar?
- How quickly do you gulp down these nachos?
- Do you even bother to chew, to taste, to enjoy, to realize what you are actually eating?
- How do you feel after the event?
- What have you learned that you were not aware of about yourself?
- Was it worth your sabotaging your new health quest? Rate it on a scale

from 10 to 0. Ten being the best experience that leads to no regrets, the food was amazing. A zero being it was crap food, what was I thinking!

- Is the emotion gone, solved, and dealt with objectively after the eating event?
- Have you taken steps to address your needs and find solutions?

This experiment is another opportunity to become more aware of your behaviors when an emotion strikes. What would your best friend's advice be in that moment?

Experiment #4: The 'let's get over it" 5 seconds rule

This is a different experiment now, we are switching gears. We are highly recommending that Experiment #4 comes after Experiment #3. I have been asking you to spend a lot of time in this book looking at your own belly button. And this was the purpose. Once you have identified your emotions and they are showing up, and you may not be ready yet with a short or long term solution, here is the 5 seconds — OK it could be 10 seconds — solution: **get over it.** Deal with it later. Do not go to the honey jar.

Repeat after me: I count 1 - 2 - 3 - 4 - 5, and then I move over. It will pass, and certainly food will not solve it. After the 5 seconds, if still struggling, you can either use the breathing technique or the visualization method, but you may be too distraught. So here is what you do. After the count to 5, if still unresolved, you can talk to yourself as if you were your best friend, or your Jiminy cricket! Here are a few examples of self-talk, you have to create your own self talk motivational sentences or quotes:

- It will pass
- It's gone already
- Food will not solve the issue. Food is not the answer
- Food will bring even more emotions
- Get over this_____ (name the emotion), it is just an emotion, it is not real. And then move on

- I am a tough girl
- I love myself, more than this cookie
- Snap out of it
- Create your own!

This is a simple method to get over a tough situation. It is not worthwhile to let the emotion pummel you and push you down into food hell. I am not saying you deal with the issue this way, and only this way, but it is a good short term solution.

This allows you to park the emotion on the side, take your distance from it, and come back to it with a clearer, more impartial, almost detached mind later. Write about it in your diary.

You will be surprised at how successful you will be.

Experiment #5: The power and joy of doing something different

Your brain is accustomed to your habits. This is the way Joy reacts, when she is sad. This is what Elizabeth does when she feels lonely. When you start to behave differently, it gives your brain a moment of confusion. The usual path is not followed, a new circuit is used. It's like being an elliptical machine aficionado, and all of a sudden switching to biking. New muscles, new move… This is what your trainer tells you to do when you feel you are stuck in an exercise rut and see no progress anymore.

Aha, says the brain, something different is occurring. So instead of cuddling your old favorite pillow while licking an ice cream cone next time you are upset, do something different. Forget about positive thoughts, mini meditation and so forth. Just do something unusual. For instance start coloring a book, or if it's still daytime, take your car and go for a walk somewhere you never went before - that little street, this unknown park in your neighborhood you never explored, this coffee shop that just opened.

You cannot go to a usual distracting habit, such as going to exercise, or calling a friend, or taking a bath. It has to be something YOU HAVE NEVER DONE before. And I am not talking about trying a new ice cream flavor! The purpose of this experiment is to surprise your brain and yourself. By doing so, you will deal with the emotion in a total new way. Your brain will forget about the emotion, because it will be too busy DISCOVERING something unknown. Your brain will register a new path in the park, views it has never seen, a coffee shop setting and menu it has never read. Of course, make a healthy choice!

Experiment #6: Experience your emotion(s)

In this experiment, we are doing the exact opposite of Experiment #5. We want you to try to simply experience your conscious phenomena without self- judging, labeling, critic, or attaching any importance to the emotion or sensation.

We are staying in the emotion. Observe your emotion. Say to yourself:

"This is just what my body and mind are doing right now, it's not good nor bad, it just is."

This will help you develop better distress tolerance and mastery of psychological experiences. This will calm you down and open new insights into your personality.

When I am myself anxious about the future, I stop in my tracks and observe my anxiety. I express the why I am anxious (already a big step) and then I look at it with a calmer eye as I write down the reasons I am anxious. As I write them down, most of them lose their sense. The situations I fear have not taken place, they are a scenario I have built in my head.

We already shared Molly's story. I feel that Molly, who wanted to stay totally anonymous to the point that I even changed major elements of her story, had to be shared earlier in the chapter.

My friends, love yourself, realize there are so many great things about you that you do not leverage in your life, that you pooh pooh or throw under the carpet. It is time for all the great assets and talents of your personality to come out and shine, explode, and come to live. It is the eclipse, in reverse. I am writing this just after the Monday August 21, 2017 eclipse. Do not let the small moon, get in the way and obstruct the huge, wonderful, life breathing and shining sunshine that is YOU!

CogniDiet® Book Club Discussion Guide

This week is all about your emotions. Try to become more rational and objective about them by identifying their sources. Not always easy I know. Again this book is not pretending to solve these issues. This chapter is here to at least give you a couple of shorter term alternatives to deflect the reaction from eating to doing something about it.

This can be a touchy group discussion, as some of you may not feel very comfortable about opening up about deep issues. Just do and share what you can. Anyhow, *The Answer is Never in the Fridge!*

- **What have you discovered about yourself this week? What do you love about yourself – please share this list. I also recommend that you ask each friend to say what they love about you. It is very enlightening and encouraging to hear other women support their friends with nice words.**

- **Have you even realized what emotions you went through?**

- **What were your first responses? Did you go for food? What type of food?**

- **Did you use the 1 to 5 snap out of it trick?**

- **Have you created a new plan to deal with emotions, short and longer term? Share if you feel like it**

- **How is the weight loss going? Challenges, new obstacles? Are you cruising? Do you need encouragement?**

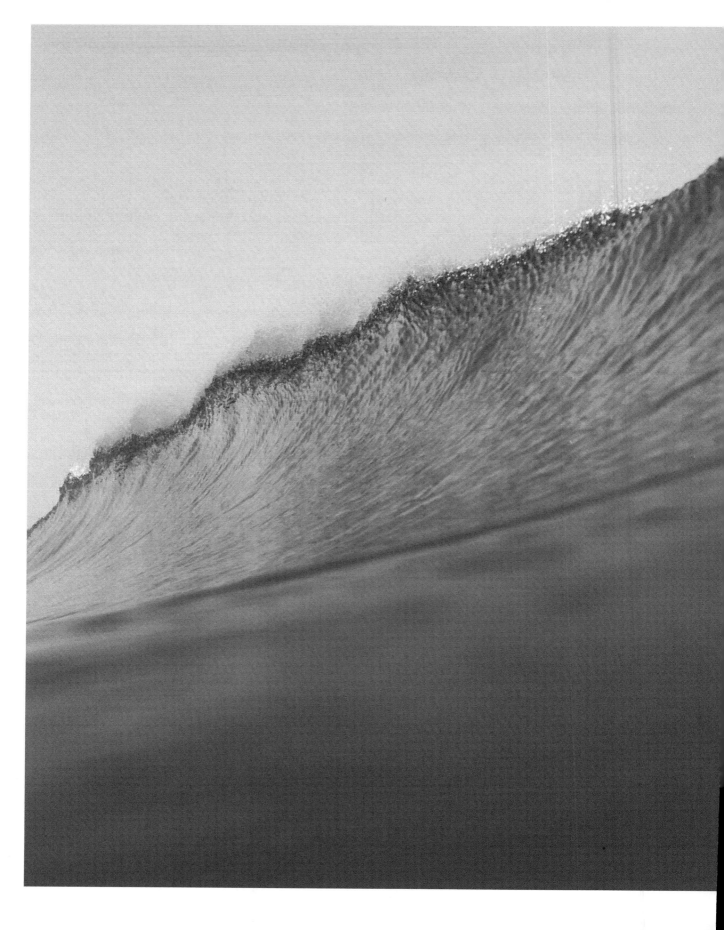

Chapter 10

Help, I'm Stuck; How to Boost Metabolism

There is always that moment when the scale is not budging anymore. Everybody has experienced that. You agonized and cried over it, suffered starvation or exercise exhaustion, self- sabotaged yourself backward, and got very frustrated. Let me be honest from the get go here. If you have lost 60 pounds, and are struggling to lose the last 5, the message from your body may be that enough is enough. Or if you are 135 pounds and have already lost 20, like one of my clients, the chances are your body is saying "STOP."

We always reach what I call the "set point." That is the weight that your body now feels comfortable at, the one you can live without being strictly disciplined or feeling deprivation. To fight your brain and body at this stage requires serious exercise upgrade, macronutrients changes or calorie cuts. But we only live once. Is it worthwhile? My advice is to stay focused on maintaining the 60 pounds loss and never letting them come back.

However, you may have lost 60 pounds and are still in a dangerous category when it comes to fat mass. You may have another 20 or 30 to go. Your desire for losing more is completely understandable. For health reasons, even more than vanity, you need to lose these extra pounds.

In this chapter I will cover and share the tools to help you unstuck your weight stagnation. You are half way, or even close to your goal but you feel there is no more ways to lose weight and you are very, very frustrated. What this chapter will not cover is anything that may have to do with a slow thyroid, pre-diabetes and insulin resistance, Type 2 diabetes or other diseases. We will give you a roadmap to check on some of these in Chapter 11, including dealing with menopause, which is a known metabolic saboteur. But we will help you with different metabolic booster tips that will help you reboot your efforts. Your mindset will be as important as your efforts.

Cogni-Tip:

I believe that the universe gives you what you want. But if your thoughts are constantly negative such as "I will never lose these next 10 pounds", or "I am incapable of being disciplined", the universe will get a NEGATIVE vibe. You need to be positive and use all the tools we gave you in this book to become positive, optimistic and visualize the next pounds vanishing from your body. The more frustrated you are, the more your body will cling on these pounds. So be POSITIVE and embark on a plan that keeps you relaxed in your mind.

There are many reasons you can reach a plateau. The body needs time to get accustomed to its new weight and diminished precious fat reserves. You have to look at your fat as a currency saving deposit that is the long term investment fund (to avoid starvation) of your body. So losing too much, too fast is like losing your retirement nest. This is why I promote slow and steady fat loss.

When you lose fat slowly, it is like you are stealing into these golden bullion reserve like a smart thief. One nugget or coin at a time, so the little greedy man upstairs—your brain—does not notice his pile of money is shrinking. However, after having stolen 30 or 60 golden coins, even slowly, there is a realization that something shifted in the body. So you need to reassure the little greedy man that it is OK for now. The plateau is a physiological and psychological good thing. A period of rest in your journey.

But you did not buy this book to wait for the greedy old man to be happy. You may not be the most patient thief, after all. What can you do to reboot or accelerate weight loss if you are in a rut? Remember that weight loss is not a linear experience. You are not going to lose two or one pound every week forever. You may lose three pounds one week and regain one the next. Your body experiences all sorts of chemical operations that are still mysterious to all of us. Why do you weight 155 pounds at 11 a.m. and without a meal, a drink, and not even peeing, you weight 157 pounds at 2 p.m.? I cannot say why, but it happens. And over the 12 week program, you will have noticed that you experienced multiple ups and down, losing three pounds one week, regaining two the next, etc. This is what weight loss looks like:

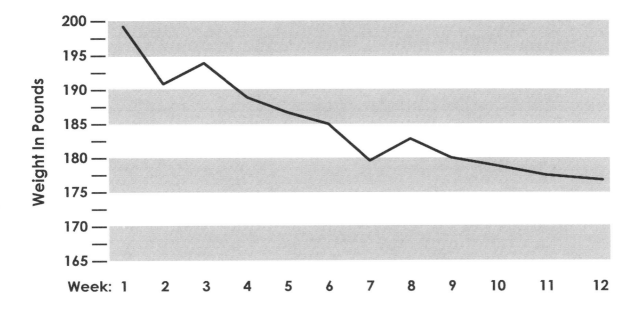

Weight loss is not linear and is not nonstop. There are ups and downs for multiple reasons. Yes it could be a week of excess, but could also be due your periods (water retention), a new medication, a life style change like an intercontinental flight trip with time zone differences, a stressful week, too much salt (again water retention), or a health issue.

In this chapter, the experiments will be sprinkled over the sections. The experiment #1 I want you to do is the following. It will help you put things in perspective, become more patient and avoid the negative thoughts of feeling like a failure because you are not losing at a steady state anymore. You have slowed down.

Experiment #1: Draw your past weight loss chart

Take a piece of paper, or go into your Excel sheets if you are familiar with it, and create a chart of your weight loss since the beginning of your quest. I advise to do this week by week, like in the graph on the previous page. If you have been losing weight for more than 12 weeks and are like in a 6 month journey, enter bi-weekly data. Then draw a line across all your results, from first data point to last one, a linear one, to show a trend. See where it leads you as far as this trend is concerned. It may give you an idea of what your next goal could be.

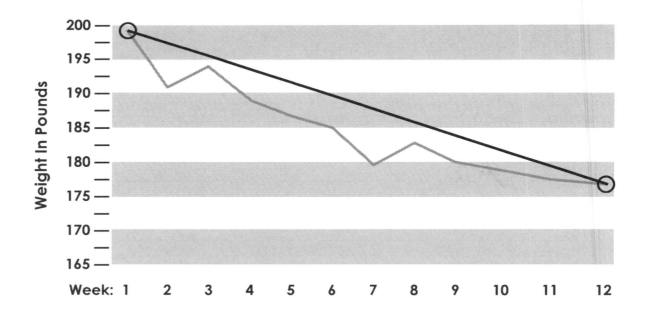

After you have done the exercise, you will realize, it may take you another couple of months to reach your next goal. Most importantly, this exercise is made to make you realize how well you did, how many ups and down you experienced and that there were plateaus! You may have reached a new plateau, again, so you need to stay the course and learn to become more PA-TIENT. Savor your past victories, write about in your diary, reflect on this journey and make a list again of all the behaviors you changed. This will put you in the right positive spirit to enter the new leg of your transformational trip.

But to go back to your reasonable question: *"What do I do if I am at a serious plateau, I have been patient enough, and I am still far from my reasonable goal?"*

Let's explore together some of the reasons that may be behind this lack of results, some-times unbeknownst of you. Nothing is more frustrating than being stuck and not knowing why, right? I hear this all the time and started a new program in September 2017 to help women over-come plateaus. Observing yourself and testing a few hypotheses we will cover, may unlock your efforts and get you back in the swing. There are a few culprits. There are short term fixable ones, which is great news. We will focus on these shorter term options in this chapter. Here is a list to start with:

- You have started to eat more again, maybe increased your calories intake without realizing

Cogni-Tip:

I heard this so many times. "Veronique, I eat healthy, I upped my veggies, I eat the good fat but I am not losing anymore. In fact I feel I am gaining a little bit every week now". **My answer: "Eating healthy has become your new SAT.** You are using the word "healthy" to give yourself permission to eat more. More "healthy "salads but maybe too much olive oil and "healthy" nuts and fruits etc. More, as in adding a coconut milk drink after dinner with turmeric because it's good for your health but adding 400 calories to your daily intake."

- You have catered to your sweet tooth again – one bite here, one bite there! You don't register the bite as calories and underestimate its impact. Remember it can be a 100 calorie bite!

- You have cut white and starchy carbohydrates and sugar, but replaced them with too much fat, even good ones, and therefore seriously increased your total calorie intake. A gram of fat is 9 calories vs. 4 calories for a gram of carbohydrates. So you are exceeding your BMR.

- You are resting on your laurels after your first 10 pound loss, which are usually the easier part of losing weight. But you have now to work a little harder to lose the next 10 pounds! And you haven't so far, let's be honest

- Your portions are still too big, maybe excessive exercising was helping negate it initially, but you just stopped benefiting from the exercise negative impact on your total daily calorie intake

- You have a mental blockage, you are afraid to lose more weight!1 Yes I have clients like this

- You are not eating enough, yes! Your body is in starvation mode

- You have destroyed your metabolism with previous multiple punitive diets, so you have reached a set point that is almost impossible to overcome (solutions coming later)

- You are too stressed, cortisol is sabotaging your weight loss efforts. It could be that there is also a short term life event that is distracting you, but you have not really realized it yet.

I will explore some practical solutions to get you back in the saddle. We will also look at supplements, certain foods or even spices that could boost your metabolism. However, let me be clear here, I am not a big fan nor a promoter of chemical metabolic boosters. Some of them are quite dangerous, even addictive, and will stop working after a while. When you stop taking them weight comes back fast. Some supplements may potentially help you but research has not established a credible clinical effect.

Let's start with the natural solutions, the ones I am most in favor of. They require that you do your homework and observe yourself over a period of at least two weeks. This is when we do Experiment #2. This experiment is meant to create an elimination list. This may help you understand why you are plateauing. It is a rather short time situation — some could be longer however—

and you have to learn to let it go. Be patient and await when the situation has abated. This experiment is meant to get practical about what you can do to separate the urgent from the non-urgent, eliminate unnecessary stress about your weight loss quest, and focus on short term solutions.

Experiment #2: Recognize and manage the temporary plateau culprits

Culprit	Solution
Terribly stressful week – or couple of weeks (new job, back to school, deadlines for a project etc.) **Important:** You know it will go away and it is time limited. It is not like a divorce which may linger for months.	Hopefully it will go back to normal. Take extra steps to relax (massage, exercise, meditation etc.). **Your action:** Take a deep breath, let it pass. Mark it on your calendar. Stay cool. Focus on maintaining your loss versus losing more.
Long flight, and jet lag	May promote water retention. Food on plane is also not so healthy (what a surprise). You have sabotaged your internal clock, it is also called your circadian rhythm. This includes eating and sleeping at unusual times. You are tired. **Action:** Wait until you recover. Drink at least your 8 cups of water a day, eat fresh and light foods, and make sure you sleep well for a couple of days.

Culprit	Solution
Too many restaurants/outings/take away in a week. But you have been such a good girl! You paid attention to what you were eating and drinking. What is happening?	In spite of your efforts to control your choices, food in restaurant is always saltier and fattier than when cooked at home. Count a 20% excess in calories. **Action:** Go on a detox – no restaurants etc. for a week or two - and adopt an especially healthy diet rich in liquids and vegetables to offset the restaurant week.
You started a new medication. There will be a difference if it is a short term or long term new treatment of course.	Some medications such as corticosteroids, anti-depressants, anti-psychotic etc. may slow down your metabolism. **Action:** Discuss this with your doctor and try to select safe and effective medications, with less impact on your weight if it is a new treatment for the long term.
You stopped exercising because you broke a foot (happened to me), had surgery or experienced any other physical impairment issue. **Attention:** It happens often in women who start to exercise later in their life. All of a sudden they may go crazy. After a few weeks, there is a torn ligament, a rotator cuff issue, a sciatica developing…	Well, well, this is unfortunate and happens more often than it should. **Action:** PLEASE if you are "a later in life" exerciser you MUST speak to a trainer, hire a trainer, and talk to your doctor before you embark on a SMART and TAILORED exercise regimen. I have seen too many accidents. **Action:** If you are a regular exerciser, and you broke a foot or had surgery, you must cut your calories to the extent you were burning them. If it was 400 calories burnt running every day, you must cut them, if you want to maintain your weight.

Culprit	Solution
The Happy and Merry Food Festival Holiday Season **It is temporary but it is the #1 reason in the U.S. for weight gain. You may gain an average of 6-10 lbs. in 3 months that "New Year Resolutions" NEVER totally offsets. The results are that you gain a couple of extra pounds every year.**	This one is so dangerous. Vigilance must be at an all-time high because everything around the Holiday Season is more sugary – alcohol, sweets, starchy vegetables, pumpkin lattes etc. or richer because it is the winter. **Action:** This book and Chapter 8 on saboteurs should really help you. The most durable weight loss results I have witnessed is when they were initiated in September/October. If you can go through the year end festivities, you can face any seasonal challenge!
A sad and difficult life event (move, loss of work, death etc.). This is different from the first one in this table where you just faced a regular more stressful week. Here we are talking about longer term.	Your energy and attention is focused on something else than your diet. Life happens. But I always say that under these circumstances, you need to be at your best in terms of energy to go through the storm and/or to help people around you. **Action:** I know it's hard. I have witnessed so many setbacks under these circumstances. Eating well must stay a priority to give you the stamina to get over this life event. Go back to the chapters on stress and emotions and use all the techniques we shared.

If at any moment, or if right now, you are going through any of the above mentioned life events, you may be rightfully at a plateau. My advice is to stay the course and focus on what is more important. Do not try to force an extra weight loss when this occurs or implement the action steps. But don't feel guilty! Guilt is a horrible saboteur.

These are temporary setbacks. You can get back on the saddle. It will pass. Yes, we can say that, but in all honesty, life always throws something at you. Week after week, there will always be something that can slow you down. There is not one week without a life challenge, I hear this all the time. So my advice is to:

- Monitor your weight, especially in these situations. I even recommend if it is a one or two-week situation to weigh yourself every day
- Lose the extra couple of pounds immediately after the event. They will go quickly
- Stay vigilant, and remember your PATs: Every day is a day where you need to pay attention.
- Develop tactics to cope with these challenging moments. Use your distractions list.

Let us now explore the other weight plateau culprits and find practical solutions to help you overcome their negative impact on your waist. I will organize them in buckets, because some of the solutions could be repetitive. Cheating with yourself is a big one, so let's start with this.

Plateau Reason #1: You are cheating with yourself — You may not know it!

You have lost a nice 13 pounds over the first week of the program and you feel pretty proud of it. You are getting slightly bored with the healthy salads and the not so exciting nuts. What would you not give for a juicy hamburger with fries followed by an apple tart with a milkshake, right?

Fall is coming and the pumpkin latte temptation is back. "Darn it!" you say next time you are at the coffee shop." The smell is so tempting, the taste is reminiscent of my youth, and the drink is so smooth, warm and sugary." So you have one. Your self-justifying SAT is, "Oh, it is only once. This will be my only one this fall." Boom, you just gained an extra 400 calories.

The next day, you are exceptionally cooking chocolate brownies (not a good idea, let me tell you) for your kids. In fact, you volunteered to bake them. Well, well, well. Here comes another SAT back. You have found a smart way to get sweets back in your life, and the excuse is the kids. You are heroic because you will only have one brownie, or so you say. But as you cook, you lick the batter, you sample the crumbles, you eat the crust, and over the next days, you may steal one or two pieces. Boom, and here is another extra 300 calories, or more, and I am nice. It could be 1,000 calories in a few days. **Even a crumble makes a difference, especially if you eat crumbles 10 times.** I know, I used to do this, chipping at the brownies my daughter Camille had baked.

That same week, you go to the restaurant with friends. You are good with the bread basket, you select a nice healthy dish. But here comes the dessert. You did not order it, but you got a spoon from your friends. You have been such a good girl for 12 weeks and have lost 23 pounds. You deserve a treat once in a while. Boom, add another 100 to 200 calories for just a few bites. Yet you feel you were a good girl because you only had a few.

Cogni-Tip:

The brain does not "count" and register the extra calories you ate over the past days. The brain just counts the calories at that moment. The brain has forgotten—how convenient— about the past brownie crumbles and batter licks etc. Even if it knows, it has conveniently decided to keep it quiet because your little brain was able to enjoy sugar again in a sneaky way.

You go to the gym the next day, because you realize you have gained one pound over the last two days. You do not really think about the extra latte, brownie crumbles, and dessert spoons you had. But combined, they may amount to an extra 1,500 calories in three days. All of these little extra cheats are made of sugar which may mean instant fat storing.

Bless you, because you went to the gym. After 1 hour of cardio, you feel like you sweat the extra fat you accumulated in the past days out, but you buy a 300 calorie protein bar at the gym. You did not need that. An old SAT came back "I need to feed my muscles proteins after exercising". This is true, but you could have added a few pieces of chicken or a sugar free protein shake. Boom, you may have lost 400 calories while running, but you regained 300 immediately! And here is the explanation for that plateau you are experiencing.

And then there is the real cheater, the closet self-sabotaging weight loss expert. You lost 10 pounds, you are very happy and proud. And because you are happy, you are rewarding yourself. You kept a survival stash of candies in your shoe closet. Every time you can, you still steal one and feel like it is only a few calories. All right, a piece of candy is maybe only 10 calories, and a wrapped chocolate mini treat may be only 30 calories. Again your brain does not make the addition. "I am eating well otherwise" is your SAT. You may accumulate an extra couple of 100's of calories in a week and do not see your scales budge. You are stagnant.

The solution is very simple. You are not losing weight anymore, and it is not due to a temporary setback as mentioned in Experiment #2. The reason is simply that SUGAR HAS MADE A SNEAKY COME BACK in your life. Cut it out NOW!

The sneaky "small bite" of sugar is the # 1 reason my clients stagnate after a while.

It is this seamless, almost unthreatening way sugar makes a comeback in your life that kills your efforts. The problem is not having an ice cream or a slice of cake once in a while. This you are conscientious of. You can deal with it.

No, I am talking about death by a thousand little arrows or little bites. Use the awareness tools you have learned in this book to stop yourself before you get that bite in your mouth girl-friends! Count to 5 always before you put something in your mouth, even a batter lick. Now let's explore the other reason you may still stagnate. I call it portion control and balanced meals.

Plateau Reason #2: The portion is still too big, the calorie intake is still too high, the macros are not balanced

Let's say you were eating 2,500 calories a day at the beginning of your journey. A higher number compared to your baseline BMR which was 1,700 with exercise, and 1,300 with no exercise. But you were totally unaware of your BMR and or just decided to ignore it, which is OK. You just started cutting some foods and calories.

You achieved an initial and impressive weight loss of 30 pounds in 12 weeks by eliminating processed food and sugar. You cut 500 calories a day and you lost 7 pounds the first week. Water was included. Then you cruised at a two- to one-pound loss a week. But after these initial 12 or more weeks, you are stuck. In reality, you are now eating 2,000 calories a day. Which is still above your BMR, plus you are not really exercising. So you scratch your head and look puzzled. You eliminated "all the bad stuff" as you say, but are not losing weight anymore.

The answer is that you are still eating too much. Your portions may still be too large. Or, there are still too many carbohydrates, and sugar, in your diet. It was easy to cut the first 500 calories. Let's face it. Now it has to become a little bit more sophisticated, thoughtful and scientific. You eliminated the sodas, the pasta and pizza at night. You tripled your vegetable intake. But you still have snacks between meals, the occasional chocolate cookie or two glasses of wine with dinner. Maybe your plate is still generously full of good and healthy foods. Maybe you still can devour an 8oz. steak with gusto.

Another reason weight loss is stagnant is my clients are compensating with too much fat. A couple of nuts here, a spoon of coconut oil in the coffee, cheese (a very dangerous one). Granted they are almost double the calories than carbs, you may have exceeded your BMR.

Here is where Experiment #3 comes into the picture. When you look at your plate tonight, please assess the calories, you may be surprised to see it is an 800 calorie plate. Make sure you include starter if any, drinks if any etc. There may still be 300 calories of rice, which is like 1.5 cups, and oh yes whole rice, but rice nonetheless. And an 8oz. steak, another 400-500 calories.

Experiment #3: If you feel that you are stuck, take action:

1. Start a food diary (again) — imperatively with calorie and macronutrients composition. I recommend an apps, it will be more reliable and less time consuming that writing and searching everything. I recommend My Fitness Pal™. Do it for three days at least. Enter everything, even the bites. Discover where you are and go back to your BMR and macronutrients percentages. Are you discovering that you still eat 200g of hard carbs a day? Or that you just eat 2,000 calories a day? Are you getting enough fat and protein? Have you added a lot of fat? What are you discovering?

2. Write a plan of action: what will you cut? And then, make a commitment

3. If you cheat because you are bored of all the same food every day, discover new recipes, make it a priority. Discover and implement at least one new healthy recipe a week

4. Go back to square one: how big is your plate at home? Draw your ideal plate and go back to assessing what it is in terms of calories. How does this plate compare to how you have been eating? Remember this plate when adding the extra fat used to cook or to create a dressing is a minimum 350 to 500 calorie plate. Adding extra fat for cooking or sauce/dressing, a piece of bread, a glass of wine make it 700-900 calories!

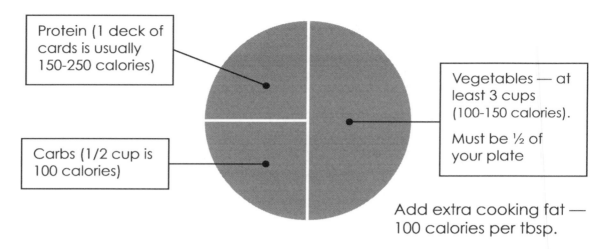

Protein (1 deck of cards is usually 150-250 calories)

Vegetables — at least 3 cups (100-150 calories).

Must be ½ of your plate

Carbs (1/2 cup is 100 calories)

Add extra cooking fat — 100 calories per tbsp.

5. Pantries/car/office etc.: Do you have sweets and pastries stashed in some locations? Have they made a comeback at home or elsewhere? Just the one bite you allow yourself once in a while, or the re-appearance of treats under the pretense that you are in control now, or it is for the kids?

Let's face it. Some of you may feel that they are in control and that they are allowing themselves, as I support, a little treat from time to time. But the danger is the sheer addition of these treats over a week. The challenge is that it usually starts with one treat a week, and then it becomes two…

Now let's look at another very different reason you may be stagnating with weight loss. And this one is related to exercise. And yes, you may be blocked because you are NOT EATING ENOUGH and are de facto starving your body. Or, you think you are exercising but are not really pushing yourself hard enough. You are mechanically doing the same old same day after day. Again, repetition does not induce calorie burning the way diversity does. You need a creative booster to your regimen. Let's start with the lady who is exercising too much and not eating enough.

Plateau Reason #3: Too much exercise, and not enough food

The good news is that you have started to exercise more. Kudos, this is a great "non-scale" victory. You should be proud of yourself. You are pretty good with food, and again, bravo. But in your quest, you may have gone too far. Impatience, zeal and enthusiasm may have become your enemies. You lost 15 pounds in 5 weeks, or more than 2 pounds a week. You are on a roll. The fat is melting. You are going to the gym 5 times a week for one hour. You listened to your trainer, and medical experts, and you combine strength and cardio scientifically. Your body is more shapely and defined. You feel more strength in your legs and you lost almost 2 sizes of clothes.

But after these initial five weeks, finito, adios, caramba, there is no weight loss anymore. You have plateaued for the last two weeks. You even went to the gym one more day and increased the intensity. You tried new exercises. But the scale is not budging. As the perfect girl that you are, you are still disciplined about the way you eat. You are very aware of what your BMR is. You are quite scientific at keeping a diary, eating fresh foods, respecting your macros etc.

However, in reality, you may have decided to ignore the fact that you need to ADD some calories back in your BMR if you are exercising hard and regularly. You were so impatient to lose weight fast.

Initially of course, you hit your body with a combined cut in food calories and a superb 400 calories extra burned 5 times a week. You are now getting maybe only a net 800 to 900 calories a day to your body, which is way too low. Remember as an average size and height woman, you should not go under a net 1,000 -1,200 calories a day.

You are underfeeding your body. So the little greedy man upstairs has put a stop to fat stealing. The body is holding on its reserves. So not only are you sabotaging your weight loss efforts, but you are also setting yourself up for altering your long term metabolism efficiency. Remember the greedy little man will want to replenish his coffers and will never forget you robbed him hard that year.

Cogni-Tip:

You need to eat more, to continue to lose weight! As bizarre as it seems, this is the reality of smart weight loss. You need to add back the calories you burn to your diet, or part of it. This is one of the hardest thing for women to accept. Try this for at least 2 or 3 weeks and see how it goes.

If it still does not work, you may have done this so many times that you have destroyed your metabolism and the way your hormones work in general. In that case, there are other solutions with metabolic boosters I will explore later in this chapter.

The second problem I have observed so many times, is women thinking they are exercising right, but not pushing their limits. This is another big saboteur for continued weight loss.

Plateau Reason #4: The not so efficient exerciser

In Princeton, which is a small city, I know a lot of people, and often see my own clients at the gym. When we explained the benefits of HIIT or interval training in Chapter 6 most of them discovered its magic and started to train this way. However many told me they were not really getting results.

I started to invite them to come and do a HIIT session with me! Yes, come with me and see how I do it. This was a huge eye opener. These CogniDiet® participants were not doing HIIT. In reality, they were very far away from it. They thought they were doing a good job. But they were not really out of breath. They were not red in the face. They were no panting and praying for the 30 minute cycle to stop. In fact they were talking to me while we were on our elliptical machines. I was secretly chuckling.

When you do cardiovascular exercise are you:

- Red in the face?
- Begging for it to stop?
- Panting?
- Sweating profusely?
- At your MHR or maximum heart rate at least several times over a period of 30 minutes to 1 hour? Go back to Chapter 6.

If your answer is none of these, then you are not really pushing yourself. And therefore you are not really reaping the benefits of exercising. If you are more like the person who walks rather than runs on the treadmill, reads a book, does emails on her cell phone, is on her cell phone on a teleconference, watches the TV screen enraptured, talks to her neighbor and does not really sweat, then you are NOT exercising. You are just being active. Maybe you do not even move really during your day, so your net benefit is just activity. It is better than nothing, but if you have already reached the maximum you can cut in foods, you are doomed to stagnate.

Going to the gym regularly for the past 15 years, and having had a trainer for so long, I have become a good observer of others. How many times did I notice a gym-goer talking nonstop to her trainer, taking her time to get on the machines, complaining about pain, stopping when it got too hard, cheating, or cruising in the back of the room during classes (poor trainers, do they push you hard or do they get sued?). If you are what I call a non-enthusiastic exerciser, how well do you think you fare when exercising? Look at yourself honestly.

Cogni-Tip:

If it is not a real hard exercise or doing intervals, it will not help you. 90% of the clients I did it with did it wrong! Get somebody to show you what a real HIIT looks like. If your health allows you to attend a high intensity boot camp, a spinning class, or a tough Zumba dance class, try it for a couple of weeks and you will reboot your weight loss. You will see results after one week, guaranteed.

Eating too much, especially of the wrong foods, cheating and not exercising smartly enough are the top reasons for being stuck. However, there can be other culprits that may be more challenging to control. Stress or a sluggish metabolism, no matter what you try with previous solutions, may still be in your way. We will now look at other tools including stress reduction, supplements and special foods, herbs and spices.

Plateau Reason #5: The stress is still getting in the way

You heard it before in Chapter 5, stress triggers cortisol, which in turn, elevates glucose in your blood, in spite of you not eating. This creates fat accumulation. You do everything right with the food and exercise, and yet you do not lose weight. The answer is that you must deal with your stress. And not just for your weight. Stress destroys your life and your health. Go back to Chapter 5 and work on it. I am insisting on this because this stress situation launches you in a very frustrating and discouraging cycle of failure. Stress impacts you and makes you feel like you will never get healthy or skinny again.

Plateau Reason #6: Your metabolism is sluggish – Let's talk about metabolic boosters

I bet some of you have either skipped the beginning of this chapter to get to what they hope are the miracle solutions. I plead that you try the earlier solutions before you get here. More often that I would like, clients rush on supplements and boosters before taking the honest approach at seriously looking at what works or not right now just with food and exercising. But it is also true, that at one point we have reached the point where we tried everything and we are still stuck. Especially as we age, our metabolism starts to slow down no matter what and it becomes harder and harder, not just to lose weight, but to keep it off.

This is where I will introduce metabolic boosters. Some are easier to implement or try than others and you may be surprised at their benefits. So here comes all the solutions:

Eat smaller meals, more often. The secret here is that when eating smaller meals you do not trigger as high a glucose spike in your blood. Even if you watch your carbs, there will always be some in your meal. For instance try on a 1,500 calorie diet to have 5 meals at 300 calories each instead of the usual 3 meals a day regimen.

But the art here is to pay attention to your macros: respect the protein, carbohydrates, fat (and real vegetables) rules.

If yours is 40% carbs, 30% protein and 30% fat, please try to adhere to this. The protein and fat linking to carbohydrates is even more important if you start to eat more frequent meals, because small meals tend to be less easy to plan, and potentially less balanced than a real meal. Are you going to eat chicken with rice and cooked cabbage in a meeting at 4 p.m. at the office?

Another challenge is that, as we have a tendency to underestimate calories, you may end up packing calories without realizing it, over 5 meals!

The other inconvenience is that it takes time and planning and may not fit within your life style. My recommendation however is to give it a try, but only if you can. If your life is too complicated, forget about it. I personally tried that and stopped. We are too busy. But it works. One alternative is to still stick to three meals a day, cut the calories to 350-400 calories a meal (not easy), and then add two smart snacks in between for 100-150 calories each.

Have a breakfast and eliminate starchy carbohydrates and sugar after 4p.m..

Cogni-Tip:

I always say to my clients. Eat like a king at breakfast, like a prince at lunch and like a pauper at dinner.

This way of eating really respects our ancestral, and still DNA imprinted energy needs. We are supposed to wake up and burn calories. When you go to sleep you do not need food. Breakfast is imperative. It sets your appetite up for the whole day.

And then, remember that carbs will not be burnt at dinner. You are going to bed. You will not be moving. You will store fat. Eliminating carbs at night is a great way to boost your weight loss. I even recommend to stop after 4 p.m. Maybe you have not been fully adhering to this early CogniDiet® recommendation (go back to Chapter 2 on sugar). Just do it for one week and I guarantee you will see results.

Eliminate processed and packaged foods — still too high in your diet. Sugars (real ones or artificial sweeteners), chemicals and preservatives contained in non - fresh food are triggering inflammation. Inflammation works against weight loss and can disrupt your endocrine system, influencing your metabolic rate. All these additives, including some contained in the environment are acting upon us as what is called "obesegens."

You may have done very good job initially by cutting calories and watching your macros. However you may also have continued to rely, for convenience, laziness or whatever reason, on processed foods. This is the next frontier for you. Remember the story about this fitness trainer who looked great but just could not lose weight anymore, She relied so much on protein powder and bars that she did not eat enough fresh foods. My biggest successes have always been with clients who started to cook seriously and became creative at bringing their own fresh food to the office. It would be a good idea for you to buy or attend a cooking class. There are multiple 30min meals and easy to cook books available on line.

Start by adding one more day, one more meal of fresh food to your weeks and you will start to notice a difference. On the contrary to other metabolic boosters this will take more weeks for you to fully reap the benefits of detoxing your body from all these chemicals. You could always get a foot in the stirrup by doing a detox week with vegetables and fruit juicing.

Respect your macros at every meal and prefer some metabolic booster foods. This one is also repetitive, but it's imperative to have a firm grasp, and control, at how you combine your foods. The plate picture we shared a few pages ago is a good way to deconstruct each meal, even a sandwich, and look at how they would fare on a plate.

An oatmeal cup will cover almost all the plate, even if not representing 600 calories, and with the plate surface being labeled as hard carbohydrates. There is almost nothing on the protein quarter, except for the few grams the milk may have offered. This is not a metabolic boosting meal. Same with a sandwich, the two slices of bread cover almost all the plate. Remember each slice of bread can be 100 calories.

You cannot have just oatmeal—almost only starches, even if they are the good long acting ones, for breakfast and then a large piece of fish, to compensate at lunch. You sabotage your metabolism. Protein takes the most energy to digest (20-30% of total calories in protein eaten go to digesting it). In general, 10% of our daily calorie expenditure is devoted to digesting foods.

You Need Balance at every Meal and Linking (Go back to Chapter 2)!

Cogni-Tip:

To the extent you can, every meal must follow a good ratio of carbohydrates/fat and protein. Try to have your 20g of protein at each meal to reach your 50-70g a day needs. Also if your macros are 40% carbs/30% fat/30% protein for instance, how do you fare meal after meal and day after day?

And yes, there are so called boosting foods, as you can read in multiple magazines. But frankly speaking I find this not too helpful. Focus on a varied and healthy diet. Fresh and balanced meals are metabolic boosters. Period.

Get enough sleep. Studies show less than 7 hours of sleep per night will make you gain weight[1]. The next Chapter, 11, will cover sleep and its overall benefits, including weight loss, at length, but when not getting enough sleep, your cortisol level gets too high therefore triggering elevated glucose in your blood. Which means fat storing.

We are talking about 7-8 hours of snooze a night. And yes, you can have a bad night and recover the next day but consistency is more important. People are not paying enough attention to their sleep, to the point I added a special class on sleep in my curriculum. It is a fact that people will eat more after a bad sleep night, with a predilection for carbohydrates. Besides, being tired will lower your ability to make logical decisions.

1: St-Onge MP, Roberts AL, Chen J, Kelleman M, O'Keeffe M, Jones PJH, RoyChoudhury A. Short sleep duration increases energy intakes but does not change energy expenditure in normal weight individuals. Am J Clin Nutr, 2011;94:410-416. PMID:21715510; PMCID:PMC3142720.

Build muscles. I will recommend that you go back to your Chapter 6 on exercising smartly. Women do not pay enough attention in general to body composition and ignore the power of muscles, being more focused on overall weight loss, no matter where it comes from. Remember that muscles occupy less space than fat pound to pound, but also burn more calories. Enroll and stick to a strength program for at least 4 to 6 weeks and you will start to notice a difference.

Cogni-Tip:

When doing this, do not focus on your scale, focus on your measurements (waist etc.) and clothe sizes. Use your pants as a measuring tool. Take pictures before and after. Strength training must be done at least twice a week. It can be combined with cardio. It can make you gain weight however because you are building muscles. This is another tough one to accept for women in general.

The 12 hour fasting diet, 12 hour diet, and so forth. Yes, there are these diets that ask you to wait 12 hours between your last evening meal and your breakfast and there is science behind it. It gives your metabolism the real rest it needs. I am myself trying to abide to this principle.

Then there is the intermittent fasting diet that may work for some people. For instance, you fast for 16 hours and then only eat within a specific 8-hour window. You only eat from noon to 8 p.m., essentially skipping breakfast, which I do not recommend. Or you only eat from 8 a.m. to 4 p.m., which is better.

Some people only eat in a 6-hour window, or even a four-hour window. You can give it a try and check some specific websites. It works. But, let's face it. Do you have the time to try this and see if it works? Is this compatible with your life style? Like the mini meals, I find this too complicated, unless you are free as a bird with almost no social life!

Now let's explore a few supplements

Honestly, you will be disappointed. I am a big "non- believer" when it comes to supplements. In my practice, besides a few useful overall supplements, I rarely recommend them.

The truth is that most weight loss boosting products sold on the market contain caffeine or green tea extracts. And they will work because of that. Or they will have phentermine, even in small doses, a stimulant associated with amphetamines. Yes that works. And it will cut your appetite, as long as you take it.

You will pay a lot of money for supplements that have not really demonstrated clinically relevant benefits. They contain multiple ingredients coming from exotic plants, but usually they will work because they contain caffeine. Caffeine is THE real stimulant that will boost the calories you burn by increasing your heart beat. Most of the supplements that will be sold use marketing tricks and dubious claims with questionable weight loss benefits will contain a caffeine, green coffee or some phentermine extracts.

1. Green tea/coffee as a drink or supplement: Yes it works. Green tea contains catechins which are metabolic boosters. Besides, green tea offers wonderful antioxidant properties. Some studies show it can boost your metabolic rate by 17% while exercising if you drink 2 to 4 cups prior to your session. 4 to 8 cups a day or supplements can help you burn an extra 50-100 calories a day? This is not an earth shattering result.

Coffee is also a stimulant. I have to say that when I drink coffee before exercising my heart rate goes up much quicker, therefore I burn more calories. However be careful, especially if you have cardiovascular diseases or are at risk. Too much will also trigger heart palpitations and extra stress. The drawback of this habit is that the minute you stop it, your metabolism slows down again. It can get you addicted.

2. Probiotics: Yes they work. Probiotics are microorganisms regulating flora in our guts. The good probiotics help with strengthening our immunity. I recommend a supplement to ALL my clients independently of weight loss goals. They have many other health advantages including a positive impact on depression and anxiety but that would require an entire new chapter or book. There are studies showing they can help with weight loss. It is believed they prevent bile salts from processing fat, which in turn and passes through your intestine, undigested. But you have to take a high amount, at least 50B CFUs per capsule (read the labels) which is the way to measure the amount of probiotics you get, and it has to contain certain strains such as Lactobacillus gasseri and rhamnosus. A particular study showed it could double your weight loss in pounds versus placebo when taking a supplement for 12 weeks. However there is controversy brewing about supplements and it is recommended to get your probiotics from kefir, yogurt or fermented foods.

3. Raspberry ketones: Some research in animals shows it might increase your metabolism. It might also affect a hormone in the body called adiponectin. Adiponectin can increase the rate at which the body burns fat and reduce appetite. However there are no real proof it works in humans.

Some of my clients reported a loss of appetite, but maybe it is just the placebo effect.

4. Garcinia Cambodia: Contains hydroxycitric acid (HCA). This chemical may prevent fat storage, control appetite, and increase exercise endurance. Again there are no real serious human studies showing it works.

5. Phentermine: Yes it works BUT it is not recommended. A stimulant similar to an amphetamine. It acts as an appetite suppressant by affecting the central nervous system. It is sold OTC and by prescription. It works, but beware when you stop, the weight will come back with a vengeance and long term side effects are not neglect able especially if you have cardiovascular diseases or take certain anti-depressants. I absolutely would never recommend this drug.

6. Leptin: This hormone regulates your appetite in your body and is, as you heard before, signaling you to stop eating. When you undergo intense and almost destructive weight loss, you are destroying the ability of leptin to tell you are full and as a consequence you may end up with an uncontrolled appetite. I have looked at so called leptin supplements. They are bogus. They are always containing caffeine or green tea. There is no such thing as a leptin supplement. This is the holy grail of pharmaceutical research.

7. The HCG diet: HCG is short for human chorionic gonadotropin. Another hormone. The promise is that HCG, when on a low calorie diet, forces and accelerates the use of your fat. This treatment is available only via prescription via injection. There are sublingual and liquid OTC versions with no proof of efficacy. The real deal is that the injection is associated with a 500 calorie a day diet. And you are surprised people are losing weight? Another very dubious, even dangerous fad. Absolutely not recommended in my world. I have seen too many clients who have been trying to recover from this starvation mode. And yes they regained all the pounds!

   There are other supplements than can be sold on their own or mixed with the ingredients cited above. These are the ones I recommend, case by case and occasionally.

1. Chromium piccolinate: It helps regulate glucose and allows for less use of insulin. It has established science. It is particularly useful if you are already facing insulin resistance. It is a well-established supplement but doses should not exceed 200mcg a day and it could damage your kidneys if taken at higher doses.

2. Magnesium: Magnesium should be taken on a regular basis for all its properties but can aid in weight loss. Magnesium is missing from our food the soil is being depleted. It may be helpful for regulating blood sugar and insulin levels in people who are overweight or obese. A 2013 study found that taking higher amounts of magnesium helps better control insulin and glucose blood levels. This same study also showed magnesium helps with bloating and water retention. It is recommended we should take 500mg a day, preferably at night.

L-Glutamine: This amino-acid can help you get your sugar cravings away. I have seen results with some clients. It does not help boost your metabolism, but it gets your insulin more efficient so may allow for less fat storing. 100 to 300mg every 3-4 hours is recommended.

Spices can also help you boost your metabolism while adding flavor and variety in your meals. They usually combine thermogenesis properties, which mean they will increase your body temperature, and I always encourage my clients to explore this avenue. Black pepper and Cayenne pepper however will deliver minimal effects:

1. Cinnamon: it mimics insulin in your blood and can help regulate glucose, therefore fat storage. It is recommended to take a teaspoon a day, sprinkled on vegetables, fruits, sauces, yogurts, puddings or even added to your coffee or tea. I know a client who mixes it with her butter.

2. Black pepper: The pungent component in black pepper called PIPERINE may fight fat by blocking the formation of new fat cells.

3. Cayenne pepper: It contains CAPSAICIN which is thermogenic. When eaten, the body needs to cool down and therefore will burn extra calories. A study from Purdue University/NIH and McCormick Spice Company by Richard Mattes, Ph.D., RD showed that on average, those who were new to eating spicy foods ate about 66 fewer calories of a macaroni-and-cheese meal on the days they ate red pepper compared to the days they didn't[2].

4. Turmeric: A study by Tufts University - Journal of Nutrition in May 2009, showed that curcumin, derived from turmeric, when given to mice and injected into fat cells inhibited the growth of new blood vessels within fat, reducing weight gain[3].
Whether this affect will work in humans has yet to be investigated in clinical trial, but the evidence looks promising. Studies also have shown that turmeric increases the flow of bile in the

2: Mary-Jon Ludy et al. (February 2012). The Effects of Capsaicin and Capsiate on Energy Balance: Critical Review and Meta-Analysis of Studies in Humans. Chemical Senses, Oxford Academy, Vol. 37, Issue 21, page 103-121

3: Ejaz,A, et al (May 2009). Curcumin Inhibits Adipogenesis in 3T3-L1 Adiocytes and Angiognenesis and Obesity in C57/BL Mice. Journal of Nutrition. 139(5):1042-1048

stomach which helps to break down fat. Taking just one teaspoon of turmeric before each meal can help your digestion break down the fat that can cause you to gain weight. We are talking about 60 to 200mg of curcumin a day. It is better taken with black pepper to boost its effect, in a hot drink or meal and with fat. Turmeric is a wonder spice that is accumulating more and more evidence it is beneficial for so many reasons, including for brain health.

We have explored all avenues to help you boost your metabolism. But at the end of the day, controlling portions, continuing to control sugar, eating more in the morning and linking carbs with protein and good fat are the best avenues when it comes to weight loss and food. And then exercise maybe your last frontier. The one you have not, but will have to tackle eventually. And remember, supplements may unlock your frustration and help but they are not miracles.

The last one! Experiment #5 for this week:

We have already suggested four experiments in this chapter. I would like to offer for this week to really ask you to try a few of the ideas we offered. A few will deliver fast results, within one week. Most strategies however, may require a couple of weeks to notice a change. You will have to learn to be patient and practice a few mental PATs that will alleviate the stress and burden that may have been triggered by your obsession and impatience at losing the next pounds too soon.

Here are the potential positive thoughts and goals you could develop to self-motivate as you embark on conquering your new plateau:

- Discipline is as important as motivation. Maybe I lost some motivation, used it as an excuse, and I need to get back to being disciplined
- I have been successful at changing my life style so far, and I will continue
- Let's enjoy my victories so far, the remaining pounds will come off when they are ready to go!
- I will take this next part of the journey as a discovery. I will find out what may really work for me!
- Let's not stress about this plateau, it is natural and to be expected. I have to learn to be more gentle with myself
- And more…

So your last Experiment #5 is to observe yourself and create your new self-motivating and very positive encouragement to tackle this new milestone. What is your next chapter motivation quote?

> ## Getting out of the plateau, my motivational quote is:

This week we will not share one story but multiple ones, because all these women got out of a rut their own way. Everybody is different. Everybody needs a different solution. The key is to realize what is in your way.

My Clients' Multiple Success Stories

Judy

At 74 years old, Judy was an initial reluctant CogniDiet® trial participant. A skeptic with a strong sweet tooth and an amazing personality! She did not count calories, did not measure macros etc. In all honesty I am not even sure she did her homework! But she knew her problem was sweets.

Her solution: The only thing she measured was her overall carbohydrates intake. She stuck to 100-120g a day. She did not use an app but watched her plate sections and became very good at estimating how much was in her bread, pasta, potatoes etc.

She also amped up her exercise. She lost 33 pounds on the clinical trial. One year later she had maintained her advantage!

Vickie

Vickie, 54 years old, did not need to lose so much. She had a tough job and a long commute. Being in retail is not easy when it comes to eating. Her problem was not quantities or portion control. Yes she liked a drink or two but that was not the issue either.

She just did not know what food was doing to her. She watched her calories like a hawk but was mostly eating carbohydrates. She was in a state of constant hunger — her own words. She ate pretzels for lunch and then got surprised she was hungry again at 3 p.m. She was completely fat averse because fat is bad, right? She literally had been starving herself for years not eating right and trying to lose weight. She has become one of our best supporters and has brought me many new clients who were impressed with her transformation.

She could not lose weight. Even at the beginning of the trial, she struggled.

Her solution: She started to eat in combinations and most importantly started to cook fresh foods and eat good fats at home. She seriously increased her fat intake, adding coconut to her morning coffee and adding salmon, olive oil, full fat dairy in her diet. This was nerve racking at the beginning she confessed! She lost 14 pounds on the trial and had lost 20 pounds when I saw her 6 months later. She has maintained that loss now over one year!

Angie (not her real name)

Angie has kids and works from home. She has a stressful, deadline driven job and spends a lot of time seated at her computer. She initially lost weight when she began cutting sweets and frequent snacks at her desk – very often triggered by stress. We knew she had to exercise more, but most importantly she had to learn to TAKE MENTAL BREAKS. She had no time to go exercise but she had a bike at home. After two weeks of plateauing and being reluctant to exercise, she finally adopted a new regimen.

Her solution: She started to take 10 to 15 minute breaks on her bike, 3 to 4 times a day, doing HIIT. She did not care how she looked afterwards because she was working from home. This was a revelation.

Low and behold, her weight loss and energy levels skyrocketed when she adopted that regimen. I remember that she was so happy and felt liberated from all her weight loss previous attempts. She not only took care of her weight but the exercise lowered her cortisol level and therefore her cravings. She lost 15 pounds over a few months.

Veronique and Paul (my husband)

Our challenge to both lose weight in 2016-17 was time. We both worked late at night. My husband is a professor and had lots of classes in the evening. Same for me. How to cook healthy foods and not resort to take outs and restaurants all the time was our challenge. Yes we are both cooks, but we had to learn to be efficient and time sensitive. Here are our solutions:

- Cook big batches of vegetables or soups on the weekend and then freeze them in individual portions. Think ratatouille. You can also freeze a meat or rice stuffed tomato, zucchini or pepper! I know, I know, you have to still cut and cook and prep but the results are worth the investment. Only a couple of hours a weekend between the shopping and the prep.

- Prepare your weekly vinaigrette as a big batch in a large mason jar (and keep in the fridge). This is one less excuse to not just toss a quick salad with pre-cut salad mix, cherry tomatoes, a few walnuts, avocados etc.

- If budget permits, you can find now all the vegetables pre-cut, spiralized, cubed, you name it in most of grocery stores, even chains. It takes only a few minutes to heat zucchini noodles in a pan frankly speaking

- Bring back food from restaurants and meetings, when it is worth its nutritional value because you can assume you only need to eat half

- Cook the night before with the goal to bring something to the office the next day

- Some vegetables are very quickly cooked such as tomatoes, spinach, even peppers, onions, zucchini, finely cubed eggplants and thinly slices anything (think ½ in. green beans, shaved Brussels sprouts or fennel etc.)

- Small cubed and oven roasted vegetables, sprinkled with spices, salt, pepper and olive oil can be ready in 30 minutes (and re-heated later)

- A piece of chicken, steak, fish, turkey, tofu can cook in a few minutes when the size is individual and reasonable

- Don't' try to be perfect all the time. It is OK to buy a pre-cooked chicken once in a while! And salad and veggie bars are available almost everywhere now

- Always have a nice and satisfying breakfast – there are nice egg muffin and crock pot oatmeal recipes now for the morning cooking averse!

By the way we both lost an extra 5 pounds in 2016. My husband has almost lost 10 pounds again in 2017, and I have lost another 3 pounds.

CogniDiet® Book Club Discussion Guide

My dear friend, we are getting close to the finish line. Some of you may have come to this chapter earlier than planned, frustrated with lack of progress. Or just impatient to accelerate the weight loss, which I am not a fan of. But it's your prerogative.

- **How is your weight? How much have you lost so far?**

- **Compare your weight loss graphs. Is the loss linear or not? Did you have hiccups? If yes, what happened? What did you do differently when your weight loss accelerated?**

- **Have you looked at your portion size, plate macros, and bites per day in between meals? Has sugar made a sneaky come back?**

- **Did you take some of the supplements mentioned in the chapter already in the past? What was your experience?**

- **How are you motivating yourself every day? Can you encourage your friends?**

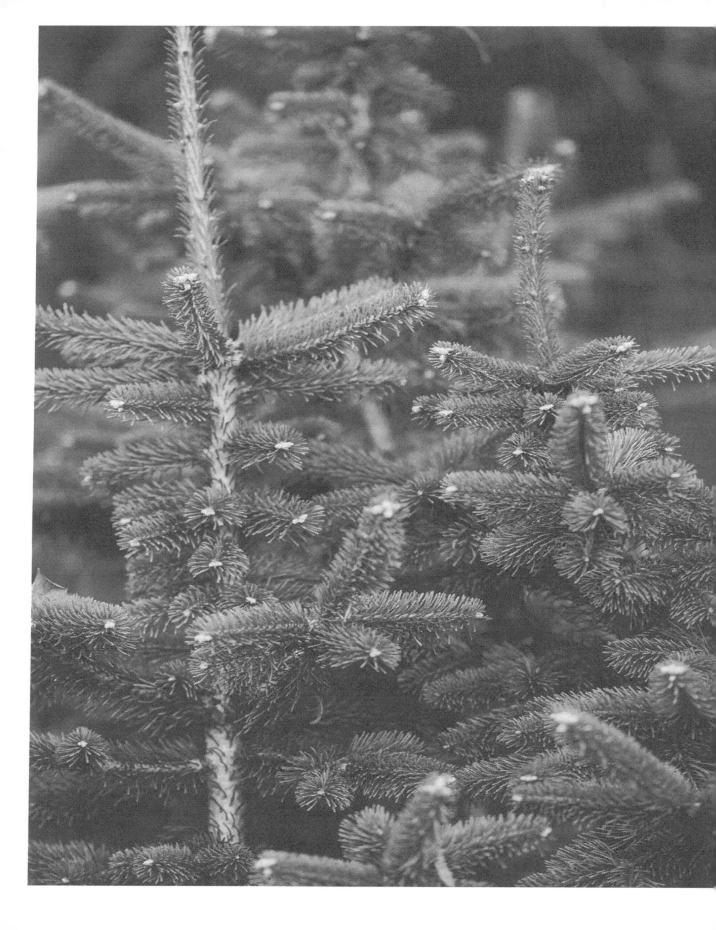

Chapter 11

I Take Care of My Health

We have now covered most of the avenues offered to you to lose weight in a natural and lasting way: leveraging your thoughts, exploiting joy and positivism to wire new happy pathways in your brain and adopting new behaviors that you love.

This chapter will cover a few health-related issues that may still be in your way as well as the benefits of sleep in weight loss and overall health.

If you don't take care of your body and your mind, no amount of weight loss will be enough to counteract a declining health. I have met too many women who were more obsessed with losing weight for vanity, than with a rising hemoglobin A1c number. And you know why? Their sabotaging thought was that "there are medications to deal with it." This is not the right approach.

I spend a lot of time explaining that after a while the problems, if not tackled, will get worse. The good news is that pre-diabetes and even early diabetes can be reversed with smart food and exercise strategies. This chapter will not cover diabetes. This is a subject in itself and there are plenty of books covering it. I do always advise my clients to regularly check not only their fasting glucose level but also their hemoglobin A1c. Too many doctors won't do it because of insurance coverage, but please insist. If you see your fasting glucose rising year after year, and getting above 100mg/dl, please check your A1c also, before it's too high. This happened to my husband.

I created a checklist of issues that most women entering their fifties could face. I always ask my clients when they work with me on a long-term basis to perform a full blood analysis with their healthcare provider and check a few extra things, especially if they struggle with weight loss stagnation and have tried everything covered in Chapter 11. Is it an under-active thyroid gland? Is it sudden menopause? Could it be a faulty digestion and food allergies? Or is it in their DNA?

I also will cover brain health—an ever-growing topic of interest as our population ages. Your brain is the most precious, commodity in your life. You cannot transplant a new brain. You cannot give a facelift to your brain, or put it under dialysis. A healthy brain is important for not only life in general, but also for weight loss. Why? All these positive thoughts and new wirings you are building in your plastic brain need nourishment as well. You are building new roads as you adopt new habits.

You want a clear mind, a relaxed brain to make the right decisions. The act of choosing a cupcake and deciding to put in your mouth requires a wiring firing in your brain. In the same vein, your ever growing desire and joy at taking your bike and going for a ride is firing pleasure neurons in your brain. You have a new pathway.

The brain is a specific part of your body with special needs. I will cover the recent findings of a study carried on with patients with early Alzheimer's disease. In this study, a multi-modality approach including food has shown the ability to slow down cognitive functions, even if it was in a very small pilot study. But it is a first. And finally, as it is growing in interest and as a new frontier for nutrition, I will briefly cover the benefits, and limitations, of DNA testing. We organized this chapter in four sections:

1. The benefits of sleep
2. A check list for your health
3. What is all that fuss about DNA tailored diets?
4. Diet and brain health

1. The Benefits of Sleep

Sleep is a much-underused ally in weight loss. It is underrated, if not widely ignored, and our society has been taking, chunk after chunk, unneglectable hours away from this deeply needed restorative time.

Sleep is your unsung hero and under-appreciated friend. In your quest to live a full life and squeeze as many hours as you can into your day, you may have pushed the boundaries of its shrinking domain. Or maybe, like many of us—including me when I was commuting to New York every day—you have a tough life juggling multiple responsibilities and having to squeeze too much in 16 hours. So your day is now 18 hours. A few of us are blessed with little need for sleep including famous geniuses and heroes, but believe me, these are a very rare breed.

Sleep is gold, sleep is a treasure, and sleep is a free occupation, no membership required. OK, I know it is not really true. One has to make a living.

While I was researching brain health and neuroplasticity, I learned so many things about sleep that I decided to develop a special workshop for my clients.

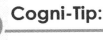

Cogni-Tip:

We need 8 hours of sleep a day. Maybe 7 hours are OK, 9 hours are even better, but cutting it to less than five to 7 hours a night has its price.

According to Wikipedia, "sleep is a naturally recurring state of mind characterized by altered consciousness, relatively inhibited sensory activity, inhibition of nearly all voluntary muscles, and reduced interactions with surroundings. It is distinguished from wakefulness by a decreased ability to react to stimuli, but is more easily reversed than the state of hibernation or of being comatose."

Multiple studies have found a link between insufficient sleep and serious health problems such as heart disease, diabetes, immune system weakening, extreme stress and obesity. In most cases, the health risks from sleep loss only become serious after years. But the short-term effects are rapidly felt.

You only use 10% of your usual energy at night while you sleep. So imagine what happens after a big dinner rich in calories...

While you dream, you are recharging your batteries. All sorts of repairing activities are going on. Sleep is when you transfer short memory to long term memory. It is also when proteins are synthesized which in turn will operate multiple functions in your body. Dreams have a role, even if still mysterious.

And you do not need studies to feel your energy, mental clarity and mood change for the worst, after even one bad bight. Thirty five hours of sleep deprivation has an impact on your ability to be involved in complex functions such as updating working memory, planning, attention, sense of time, dealing with novel situations, and verbal fluency.

When I am tired, I mean really tired, I start to mix my languages. I want to speak in English as usual, but I start to speak Dutch. It's as if my brain is short-circuited. Or I have a hard time finding my words. I feel as if I am a little bit drunk and foggy brained. Studies show that continued sleep deprivation, used as torture, leads to hallucinations and delirium and eventually death.

There are five different stages of sleep, from very light to very deep. Stage five is called the REM (Rapid Eye Movement) stage. It is when dreams occur. But it is in stage three and four, just before REM, when you are in the deepest sleep, that the most restorative operations take place. These five cycles occur several times during the night.

There is a proven link between REM sleep and the repair of cognitive functions. Activity in parts of the brain that control emotions, decision-making processes, and social interactions is drastically reduced during deep sleep, suggesting that this type of sleep may help people maintain optimal emotional and social functioning while they are awake.

But What about Sleep and Weight Loss?

In one research project, subjects were restricted to four hours sleep per night. After only a few nights their metabolism had shifted, and their muscles were less efficient in absorbing glucose from the blood (www.ncbi.nlm.nih.gov/pmc/articles/PMC1991337/). Losing out on sleep can make fat cells 30 percent less able to deal with insulin, according to a study in Annals of Internal Medicine (www.annals.org/aim/article/1379773). In another study simulating the effects of a disturbed sleep patterns of shift workers on 10 young healthy adults, three of them had blood glucose levels that qualified as pre-diabetic after three days.

Recurrent sleep deprivation in men increased their preferences for high-calorie foods and their overall calorie intake. And women who slept less than six hours a night or more than nine hours were **more likely to gain 11 pounds (five kilograms) compared with women who slept seven hours a night.** Other studies have found similar patterns in children and adolescents according to Donald Hensrud, M.D., author of "The Mayo Clinic Diet". Even from a CBT perspective, one should be disciplined about going to bed and getting up at the same time. Consistency is crucial for developing a beneficial sleep pattern.

Part of the problem with lack of sleep is behavioral. Because you are tired, you will not go to the gym, or will stay on the couch. Because you are tired, your resistance to food temptations will be lower as well.

The other problem is when you do not sleep enough, leptin levels gets too low. Remember, leptin tells you that you are full. Also, cortisol levels get too high. The results are that you will eat more with a predilection for carbohydrates.

Therefore, to not gain weight, you need to get your sleep. I am myself pretty disciplined about sleep; you could call me a bore or a granny. I don't care. I want to jump out of my bed refreshed and energized every morning. Besides having the discipline to go to bed on time to get your eight hours, here are a couple of tips if you have a hard time getting to bed. Bedroom decoration, pre-sleep activities and foods and drinks all have an impact on the quality of your sleep.

- Your bedroom must be uncluttered. It is not an office, it is not a TV room. This can and will impair the quality of your sleep by impacting the feng shui factor of the room. Every unnecessary object is an energy stealer. Computers and TV or phone screens emit electric waves that will sabotage the quality of your sleep. A welcoming and calm bedroom will appeal more to you because it enhances the value of sleep.

- You need dark curtains to mask the light, a comfortable mattress and pillows, and the right temperature, ideally between 60 and 67 degrees. The best colors for your walls, according to research are blue, green and lavender to induce calm.

- You need to relax before going to bed, it will allow you to fall asleep faster. A horror or violent movie before bedtime, or video games will stimulate your brain too much. For instance, take a hot bath, do yoga or meditate.

- Do not embark on cardiovascular exercise before bed, it will get your metabolism revved up and will prevent you from falling asleep.

- No big meals, or too much alcohol before sleeping. The alcohol may knock you down initially but it will wake you up a few hours later.

- No caffeine or stimulants at least 7 hours prior to bed.

Then there are the other saboteurs, the ones that will even impact the quality of your dreams:

- Going to bed angry or with a problem on your mind. Deal with it, let it go and go to bed appeased. Several tricks can be used. You can write the thought or feeling in a journal and then let it go. Some people put a little paper in a "worry box," because rehashing doom scenarios and worries in your bed will not help. I know it is easier said than done. But you have learned to work with your thoughts. Please try to postpone the worry to the next morning.

- Working in bed. You bed is for sleeping. Working in your bed conveys a sense that the bed is an office extension. Reading a nice book is fine however. If you have to do emails, get in a chair in your bedroom or elsewhere, but not in the bed.

Cogni-Game:

My last advice, because I believe in the power of dreams, is to either pray if you are religious, or before you close your eyes, visualize your new self and summon the universe to bring it to you. Thoughts of happiness, gratitude, joy and hope will percolate into your dreams and will help you fall asleep at peace with yourself. And imagine symbolic pounds of fat going into the ether as you sleep. Sleep one year and you could shed a few extra pounds, or at least not gain extras. You just read it. It could be one extra pound a month!

2. A Checklist for Your Health

Some of your most important weight loss potential saboteurs include a slow thyroid, menopause, a not-so-well functioning digestive system or liver, and diabetes. Lack of certain minerals or vitamins can also hinder weight loss efforts.

I am not going, in this chapter to cover all health aspects pertaining to a woman. Of course do your mammograms, pap smears and pelvic examinations regularly. Do your colonoscopy. Watch your heart and take good care of yourself. Take care of your mental health. Watch your bones after menopause. Go to your gynecologist.

I will focus on weight related issues. Having so many clients that are peri-menopausal, I always give them a check list of what they need to discuss with their doctors. Checking your health is good practice in general. Certainly, it will benefit you to do it sooner than later if you feel stuck with weight loss in spite of your best efforts.

A. The thyroid gland: A slow thyroid gland or underactive thyroid will slow down your metabolism. On the contrary an overactive one will help you stay fit. Some of us are blessed with very effective thyroid glands. The challenge is that, as everything else, its efficiency will go down with age. Your thyroid gland is an endocrine gland located in your neck. This gland plays a crucial role in the body by producing the hormones T4 (thyroxine) and T3 (triiodothyronine). There is a very complicated cascade, like a ballet, of subsequent activities that help regulate your metabolism, which means getting the highest energy possible from food and burning fat at the maximum rate. Your thyroid also plays an important role in breathing, heart rate, menstrual cycles, cholesterol, and more.

Some of the symptoms of an underactive thyroid are trouble sleeping, fatigue, depression, weight gain, and heavy periods. The thyroid gland function decreases with age. Ridha Arem, M.D., an endocrinologist, who currently runs the Texas Thyroid Institute, at the Texas Medical Center in Houston is the author of a book I recommend: "The Thyroid Solution" which explains what the problem can be, its impact on your health and diet and treatment solutions.

Many women may suffer from a slightly underactive thyroid because they have a history of yo-yo dieting. They have given a hard time to their thyroid for too long, and the gland is tired. Interestingly women represent the vast majority of patients with thyroid problems. Finally, women tend to internalize stress, which also affects their adrenal, brain, and thyroid functions, resulting in increased cravings for sweets and simple carbs to provide instant energy and feel- good hormones

If you are in doubt, ask your doctor for a thyroid test. I recommend going to an endocrinologist rather than your primary care as the devil is in the details with all these T hormones. Plus they will look at your other hormones, such as cortisol and the sex hormones associated with menopause. In no case, do buy over the counter so called thyroid boosters. They can wreak havoc on your organism and mislead test results. A thyroid gland issue is a serious issue. Talk to a doctor.

B. Menopause and sex hormones: As we become peri-menopausal everything changes as we gradually lose our beneficial sex hormones. Yes, periods are gone, good riddance. But hello bad nights, weight gain, hot flashes and general mood swings. Not fun. I experienced brutal menopause at 43 when they took my ovaries out overnight. So I did not benefit from a gradual slow down as it happens usually. I experienced a shocking withdrawal. I will qualify it as HELL.

Honestly, I turned to hormone replacement therapy or HRT, because as an executive I needed my sleep. Sleep deprivation was my biggest issue. I could deal with the hot spells and the dry skin. I took HRT pills for a couple of years, then started to wane off and ended completely after a couple of years. To encourage you, even without any HRT after a while, I have lost weight, I sleep well, and my skin is fine. The sex drive is what it is! So my message is that it is manageable over the long term, you just have to learn to navigate through an initial rough patch. But this book being about weight loss, let me explain why we gain weight at menopause. Darn it, it is so unfair. When menopausal, all sex hormones levels start to go down, with consequences:

- **Estrogen:** Because your estrogen level goes down, and by the way the ovaries continues to deliver them for a very long while, just at a lower and lower level, your body is looking for another source. And another source for estrogen is fat cells! What a surprise. What your tricky body does then is to create and keep more fat cells, to release estrogen and compensate for the failing ovaries. Your body learns to convert more calories into fat, in order to increase estrogen production. This means weight gain. This is one of the reasons you gain fat around the abdomen when you get menopaused. Crazy unfair and frustrating. It is harder to get rid of fat as we age.

  Solution: There are two major strategies to work against abdominal fat: cutting carbohydrates and sugar and doing interval training. A MUST for the post-menopausal woman.

- **Progesterone:** This hormone level also goes down. Low levels of the hormone do not actually cause you to gain weight, but instead cause water retention or bloating. So now you are getting fatter and bloated, how nice!

  Solution: Avoid salt, processed food – rich in salt - and drink at least 8 to 10 cups of water (not seltzer, tea, coffee or soda) a day.

- **Testosterone:** Yes, we have some of it too and for some of us, more than others! Testosterone works to build and maintain muscle mass among other things. These muscle cells work to burn calories in your body and cause a higher metabolism. When you enter menopause, you lose muscle mass and therefore lower your metabolism. This also results in weight gain.

  Solution: Build muscles and do strength training at least twice a week.

HRT has been a controversial treatment that needs to be addressed with your physician. A large study published in 2012 showed increased risk for breast cancer. There are also more natural and local treatments besides a pill, including creams to enhance your vagina's lubrication, which is another side effect of menopause.

Besides HRT treatments, supplements to alleviate hot flashes can help and include soy and black cohosh. The soy molecule mimics the estrogen molecule, but I do absolutely not recommend soy if there is a history of breast cancer in your family. I say: avoid eating soy, a plant that is also heavily genetically modified. The herb black cohosh can work for hot flashes, but with a wide variety of responses. It is a rather safe option however that you can try.

The reason for this section in this chapter is to alert you about the consequences of menopause and encourage you to take the best action for the control of your weight. Please eat less, avoid starchy carbohydrates and sugar, embark on strength training to build muscles and absolutely do interval training or HIIT at least 3 times a week.

C. An optimal digestion: Digestive enzymes, food intolerances and allergies: Digestive enzymes will also go down as we age. We have an enzyme supply at birth that we deplete over the years. These enzymes are the little miracles that cut all the food in smaller pieces for us to assimilate them in our body. They cut the protein chains into smaller pieces called amino acids that are then used for certain functions. Combined with probiotics, I have seen some serious digestive improvements in clients.

Not digesting foods well means these foods may be going through your digestive tract unable to be assimilated fully, creating deficiencies in nutrients including vitamins and minerals. This in turn is not only not good for your health but may sabotage your weight loss efforts. To be noted that enzymes are specific to carbohydrates, protein or fat. So you may need different types. You may notice that you are bloated or not feeling so well after a pancake breakfast, or more like after you ate a very fatty meal.

You may benefit from enzymes if you feel symptoms such as constipation, gas, bloating or diahhrea. If you have low stomach acids or are taking an antacid, you should take extra enzyme supplements.

Make sure when you buy enzymes that they are of the utmost quality. And are from vegetal origin. Look for fillers such as magnesium stearate, maltodextrin, silicon dioxide and other additives that should be avoided. I bet some of these enzymes will be familiar to you: bromelain (a source is pineapple), papain (a source is papaya), amylase (especially for carbohydrates), cellulose and lipase.

Many people confuse them with probiotics. They are often sold together. There is no real way to know what you need. You need to find out how you react to certain foods. But to simplify your life, and once over 50, I recommend you take a general combination of enzymes that will cover carbohydrates, proteins and fats digestion.

And finally check your liver. Remember the fatty liver story. It can only be detected with a CAT scan but your doctor can check your liver enzymes and by doing so, see if something is not working well. And your liver loves a good detox, such as no alcohol for instance!

D. Food allergies and intolerances can also be tested now either via DNA testing, allergy battery testing with an allergy specialist, or via plain and simple self-observation.

Gluten intolerance, not be confused with celiac disease or irritable bowel syndrome or IBS, is a trendy one. It is an intolerance, not an allergy and not a disease. The food industry has jumped on that craze. There is controversy about what gluten intolerance really is. Is it gluten really or is it the way our cereals have been genetically modified and completely submerged with dangerous pesticides? Again this is another book. And by the way, gluten intolerance can also be detected with DNA testing.

Gluten is not just contained in wheat, rye and barley. Gluten is used as a food additive by the food industry in multiple processed foods usually as a thickener or an element to add some chewiness. Here are a few foods that contain gluten (funny how so-called gluten intolerant avoid all carbs but still eat ice cream!):

- Soy sauce
- Most of condiments
- Mustards
- Dressings
- Cheese spreads
- Most of industrial ice creams and yogurts!
- It is added to almost ALL prepared foods such as frozen or canned preparations meals including meats, soups, vegetables, beans, potato spuds...
- Gluten is added in some chewing gums, fruit drinks, protein shakes, fake seafood and some meat pates as it is used as a binder

You must become a label detective. And 80% of my so called gluten intolerant clients eat some of the foods mentioned above with no problems!

The second danger I want to mention if you go gluten free is that most of the gluten free pasta, pastries or cookies are made with rice or corn flours. They are cheap, over-processed flours which possess a very high glycemic index! So, yes, you may be eating a gluten free cookie, but this does not mean it is carb free! And it may be awfully expensive. Better options, although more expensive, are nut flour such as almonds or rarer cereals such as spelt, amaranth or millet flours. These ingredients will make for a higher quality gluten free product.

E.Vitamins and minerals: I am not a big supporter of multi-vitamin complexes. The reason is that tablets or capsules are huge and difficult to digest. This is because the companies try to put so many components together. You may also end up with too little of what you really need. But some of you maybe really not getting enough via your food. My advice is to check your essential ones with your physician ASAP.

What I will ask you to do is ensure you test:

- Vitamin D levels, which are important for your bones amongst other things.

- Some vitamins and minerals that are important if you are highly stressed and they are vitamin C (cannot be checked but take at least 1,000mg a day), vitamins B (especially B12 and B6) and magnesium.

- At least once or twice a year, ask your doctor to check these: iron, calcium, potassium, zinc, copper, selenium. It may be extra cost in some cases but it is worth the investment.

3. What Is All That Fuss About DNA Tailored Diets?

23andMe®, and other DNA general health and ancestry testing kits, are now available without a healthcare practitioner involved, for you to test yourself. You will not only discover some of your ancestry genes, but also some other health and nutrition related genes such as lactose or gluten sensitivities, Alzheimer's disease, cancer, Parkinson's etc. The most important benefit of DNA testing from a health perspective is to educate you about your risks. A well informed person is better equipped to take pro-active measures to prevent or delay the onset of these diseases or health issues. It is not easy to swallow that you are at risk from breast cancer, but it is better to know!

Other companies offer even more in-depth nutritional testing. The new frontier in nutrition will be DNA based nutrition, also known as nutrigenomics. Companies are already sprouting, offering tailored prepared meals following a special DNA test and metabolic test. You can discover your ability to assimilate vitamins, minerals, carbohydrates and fats. You will know if you are lactose or gluten intolerant. You can also discover some fitness related genes such as endurance, ability to build muscles or resistance to pain!

Some of us are better equipped at dealing with gluten, or processing certain vitamins. You may be chronically deficient in iron, or you may not digest certain fats so well. You may have a sugar tooth or a slow metabolism gene.

I am a believer in DNA testing and in our office we provide testing with Nutrigenomix®, a

Canadian based company that looks at 45 genes, related to nutrition, physical stamina and pain tolerance. I did the test first and discovered a few things that surprised me, and some I was intuitively aware of. For instance, I do not assimilate vitamins B well, so I am taking a supplement daily now. I also have a gene that affects how much coffee I can take and I should limit my intake to 2 cups a day. I find this very useful general information in the sense that it has made me more disciplined about for instance taking some supplements. This will enhance my health overall.

It has also made me an even more conscious eater. I did not know I had a gene that made me slightly intolerant for gluten and not the best at assimilating carbohydrates. So I am paying even more attention than before. Not that I eat so many carbohydrates anyhow. But since I have known that, and to my chagrin, I have cut even more on the French baguette, a staple from my childhood - it is the high gluten content that makes it so chewy! Besides it is a white carb right! So I went from cheese and baguette once a month to once a quarter. True. Tough to be French!

I also discovered I have a slow metabolism, thank you my genes, how unfair is that. I have cut my portions and have lost another 5 pounds in the last 6 months, just because of that.

There is, however, a big caveat with genotyping. Years of extreme dieting or just unhealthy eating habits may also alter your hormones, fat volume and metabolic processes. A person who did not have the gene that may promote sugar addiction, when tested, may still have become addicted to sugar because of habits formed over the years. The brain will become addicted, no matter your genes, if you eat too much sugar. It is just like some of us will become addicted quicker and/or stronger.

I want to be clear. Genotyping is only one part of the story. Speak to your healthcare practitioner and/or nutritionist and take a test, it is also a few hundreds of dollars, and different companies provide it now. Discuss the results with them. You may not understand the meaning of all the results. They will help you design a plan.

Cogni-Tip:

Do not use the DNA results as an excuse, to eat more sugar because you have the bad gene (what a beautiful SAT), or to not exercise so hard because you have a low threshold to pain (hello SAT again). Use it positively and to your advantage.

4. Brain Health

Remember my story. I experienced first-hand what a brain in trouble can do to your life: overall gloom and doom, depression, anxiety, panic attacks, lack of focus and concentration. So much fun to live like this! And I am not the only one, by far.

Most of us nowadays live a rather stressful life. Really, who can say they have no stress? And you now your brain does not like that. Plus your little brain is so busy every nanosecond making decisions, creating new pathways, storing memories, learnings new things and just trying to be happy.

So what does your brain need to function well and be happy? It needs (you should be able to fill in that list by now):

- Sleep - As you read earlier
- Balanced foods – Your brain needs a balance of proteins, good fats and good and fresh carbohydrates
- Exercise to get the endorphins firing and the blood flowing
- Relaxation to promote alpha waves that have proven stress, anxiety, and pain relief properties. It also promotes memory strength.
- Joy. We need to laugh, we need to socialize, and we need to have fun.

Besides These Elements, There Are a Few Supplements Your Brain Really Needs:

Brain Functions	You need
Short term memory	Folate, Vitamin B12, Vitamin C, Choline
Problem solving	Riboflavin, Folate, Vitamin B12, Vitamin C
Dementia	Thiamin, Niacin, Folate, Vitamin B12, Zinc
Cognition	Folate, Vitamin B12, Vitamin B6, Iron
Degeneration of brain tissue	Vitamin B6
In general	Omega 3, glucose, oxygen, atioxidants such as flavonoids and carotenoids, curcumin, water and sleep

This is why you keep on hearing me repeating again that a vitamin B complex must be a staple in your armamentarium.

Prevention of Memory Loss in Alzheimer 's Disease

A 2015 study has made headways recently and a book has been written about it. A new protocol has been created. It is called The Bredesen Protocol (www.drbredesen.com/thebredesenprotocol).

Dale Bredesen, M.D., is a physician and a neuroscience researcher. He is internationally recognized as an expert in the mechanisms of neurodegenerative diseases such as Alzheimer's disease (AD). He is the Augustus Rose Professor of Neurology, director of the Easton Center Institute at the Buck Institute for Research on Aging at UCLA.

He studied reversal of cognitive decline in, yes a small, but nonetheless very encouraging study. The study has been published in Aging 2015. It is the first to suggest that memory loss in patients may be reversed — and improvement sustained — using a complex, 36-point therapeutic program that involves comprehensive diet changes, brain stimulation, exercise, sleep optimization, specific pharmaceuticals and vitamins, and multiple additional steps that affect brain chemistry. It does not include specific prescription drugs for AD.

The reason I am sharing this is because what is promoted in this protocol is exactly what a healthy, nutrient-rich and common sense diet should be. Period. We should all eat like this, every day, to prevent rapid aging and not just AD. We need it to promote better health and not just to improve cognitive functions.

Dr. Bredesen's approach was personalized to each of the 10 patients in the study, based on extensive testing to determine what is affecting the brain's plasticity signaling network. His therapy included – this is not an exhaustive list:

- Eliminating all simple carbohydrates (it means all the white stuff), gluten and processed food and eating more fresh vegetables, fruits and non-farmed fish. Familiar advice isn't it?

- Meditating twice a day and beginning yoga to reduce stress. Again makes sense, right?

- Sleeping seven to eight hours per night (up from four to five for his patients)

- Taking melatonin (to sleep), methylcobalamin, a form of vitamin B12, vitamin D3, fish oil and coenzyme Q10 (aids in basic cell functions) each day

- Fasting for a minimum of 12 hours between dinner and breakfast, and for a minimum of three hours between dinner and bedtime

• Exercising for a minimum of 30 minutes, four to six days per week

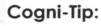

Cogni-Tip:

Here above is described the healthiest, most natural diet. You have heard it before in this book. Stick to that diet and not just for your memory.

Nine of 10 participants, displayed subjective or objective improvement in their memories beginning within three to six months of this protocol. So be patient!

Six patients had discontinued working or had been struggling at their jobs at the time they joined the study; all were able to return to their jobs or continue working with improved performance, and their improvements have been sustained. One patient who had been diagnosed with late stage Alzheimer's did not improve. The findings are published in the current online edition of the journal "Aging".

The results are anecdotal yet encouraging. A bigger, controlled clinical trial is needed. But this study has made huge waves. It means that a broader multi-functional approach, rather than a single drug treatment, may be potentially more effective for the treatment of cognitive decline due to AD. By the way weight loss was also observed.

Cogni-Tip:

(no pun intended!): So my dear friends, eat well, sleep well, move well, think well, and you will improve all your health indexes including your cognitive functions! And oh yes, also lose weight.

This concludes this chapter and I would now invite you to discover Joyce's story. She did not do well on the clinical trial, but she unlocked her issues by visiting her doctor and then a miracle happened.

Joyce's Story: A Failed Trial and a Successful Story

Joyce (not her real name) is a lovely petite blonde with a sunny and charming personality. She really struggled on the clinical trial and definitely there was a sweet tooth issue there. She did not need to lose that much to be honest. She was just a little bit chubby around the waist.

She started to exercise more and become more conscious of her choices by the end of the 12 weeks. She felt bad at the end of the program and said "I feel like I let you down." She had lost two pounds. Interestingly the last chapter we covered was this one and she became very interested in her thyroid gland. She knew everything else was OK. She was pretty healthy.

I hear this often in my clients' voices. They have hopes and expectations that maybe the thyroid gland laziness is the answer to their prayers. "I hope my thyroid is the reason I am stuck." And it can be very true. It is a very frustrating ordeal to work hard and observe no results in spite of heroic diet and exercise changes.

When I saw her for the 6 months follow up in July 2017, she looked even better and she was radiating with happiness. She had lost 8 pounds (she is a petite woman and did not need to lose more than 8-12 pounds). She had been to see her physician after the trial and had checked her thyroid gland. And she was right, she had a lazy one. She started to take some medications and saw a very rapid difference in energy and metabolism. That boosted her self-confidence and enthusiasm like a rocket. I just saw her again in December 2017, one year post trial, and she has now lost 12 pounds!

I am sharing this story today because I don't want you to feel bad if you are stuck and know you are trying everything to succeed. The worst you can do is not talk to anybody about it, not do some research or go and see your doctor.

- Is it my constant stress? You can check your cortisol level but it will only give you a "time in point" reading. The best way is to observe your weight evolution and your stress level and then go back to Chapter 5 or visit an endocrinologist who could also find you adrenal glands fatigue. Or go see a professional who can help you with stress reduction, with medications or not.

- Is it my thyroid? Check with your doctor.

- Am I allergic/intolerant to some foods? Do the tests with your physician.

- Am I insulin resistant? Please, please, not only check your fasting glucose but also your A1c with your healthcare practitioner.

- Is it my lack of muscles (time to check with a specialist or at the gym)?

- Is it my genes? Do a DNA test, it is eye opening and empowering!

Joyce was elated. She felt she was not alone anymore. In the class, she shared her struggle and frustrations getting on the scale every morning and not really seeing results. She told me she cried sometimes. She wanted to stop the trial. She did not know what to do anymore except starving! She had a sense of injustice and unfairness.

She finally felt vindicated because she — her words — looked like a failure on the trial witnessing her friends losing 15 pounds or 33 pounds. And she knew during the last 6 weeks of the trial that she was really a good girl, using her PATs, de-stressing, exercising and cutting sugar, all this over the Holiday season.

There is a lot of power in KNOWING what is going on in your body. I urge you to be curious about your health, stay informed, read a lot, attend conferences and get seriously involved with your treating physician when it comes to anything you feel is not right.

Do your yearly physical, check your symptoms, learn to test your breasts, observe your periods and feces (not joking, there could be blood in them). Please do your colonoscopy after 50! You can even play with a glucose monitoring device and see how you are doing on your own. You can check your blood pressure, you can check your heart rate after running. So many things you can do. I have done them all.

....

This Week's Experiments

Experiment #1: Take one health related action

This week, decide what matters more to you. Is it that you are undergoing menopause, and you feel you want to discuss hormonal support with your physician? Is it that you want to test your A1c again, or that you have elevated fasting glucose but your doctor did not see fit to check your A1c yet? Or is it that you have been willing to splurge in one of these DNA tests? It does not have to be just one thing. But remember endless to-do lists. I'd rather you prioritize and take one step at a time.

Or create a list of priorities based on your suspicions. A first step is important. It could be your thyroid gland like Joyce. But she knew everything else was OK. Do your check list. You could suspect a problem with your thyroid but maybe also experience adrenal fatigue. Once you see your doctor for your next physical, make sure you cover all the topics you want covered and get all the tests needed. Be assertive and demanding and do not take NO for an answer. I know insurance companies are difficult but sometimes your healthcare practitioner may be too busy to fight for you!

MAKE ONE (or 2 or 3) DECISION. IMPLEMENT.

Write: This week I will _____.

And just do it!

But write here what you will do with the results, good or bad. In fact what will be your next steps?

Experiment #2: Examine, sort out, prioritize, eliminate, and question all these supplements you are taking

You were already, or have now become a much savvier health expert. Your health quality — the attention you pay to it — and nutritional IQ have grown tremendously, or so I hope. You may or may not take vitamin and mineral supplements yet, or you may take too many.

Ask yourself these questions for each supplement, or go and discuss it with your physician or pharmacist (free!):

- Am I taking the right amounts?
- Is this a good quality brand?
- Am I missing anything in terms of supplements?
- Is there a supplement I take that I may not need (if prescribed by your doctor, speak to him/her first). Maybe this has been going for a while, do I still need to take this vitamin A? I don't even remember what for!
- What is the expiration date on this package? These vitamins E have been in my cabinet for two years.
- Am I taking these supplements at the right time of the day, with or without food? It could negate some of the efficacy.

This experiment will help you either become more serious and disciplined about taking your supplements and treatments or will help you streamline your regimen and clean your cabinet. Focus is of the essence.

Experiment #3: Am I really gluten or lactose intolerant? And if I don't know, let's try a week without gluten or dairy!

You have seen the list of products that contain gluten. Are you still eating some, and are they still in your kitchen cabinet? If you are, or think you are gluten intolerant, maybe it is time to revisit this status. Or maybe do a little experiment!

1. You do not believe you are gluten intolerant (you could conduct the same experiment with lactose)

Eliminate all gluten containing products and foods from your diet for one week. Notice how you feel. The following are symptoms associated with gluten intolerance. Did you experience them? If yes, how do you feel after one week gluten free? Did they disappear?

- Bloating, diarrhea, gas
- Fatigue or brain fog after a meal containing gluten
- Chronic fatigue

- Chicken skin on your underarms
- More serious: diseases associated with gluten intolerance such as celiac disease, IBS, autoimmune diseases, hormonal imbalances for instance. If you have these diseases, avoid gluten!

For lactose intolerant folks, there is also this belief that it is not the lactose so much but the source and quality of the dairy that matters. Have you tried pasture and organic raised milk or yogurt? Have you tried sheep or goat milk yet (it has to be pasture fed and organic)? Just try. You may discover that you don't experience such discomfort. So maybe unless it was confirmed via an allergy test, that you are not seriously intolerant!

2. You are gluten intolerant but may have not been so good at eliminating sources because…

Read your labels… Assess how much you may have eaten unbeknownst of you. Re-assess your status, are you really gluten intolerant?

Experiment #4: Spend one or two weeks eating and living like Dr. Bredesen's patients

Use his protocol, as far as eating, relaxing and exercising is concerned. For one week or two, what have you noticed? Do you feel more energetic, smarter and more performant overall from a memory, concentration and work endurance point of view? Could you work one more hour today? Maybe two?

If you live with an aging parent at home, why not adopt this protocol and observe how your cherished mom is doing? Maybe she won't forget the milk in the garage or put salt in her coffee anymore? Maybe it's time to speak to her doctor about the Bredesen protocol?

This experiment will reinforce your beliefs and proven benefits of eating healthy and naturally. **If you don't do it for your weight, do it for your brain!**

Experiment #5: Learn to read your labels

One of the most beneficial benefit I have seen in our program, besides weight loss, is the complete change of behavior of my clients when it comes to label reading. They now question everything. It has really allowed them, without becoming food snobs, to eliminate a lot of the processed stuff they were eating and/or to start to buy better and healthier options. It has made them, even for the penny pincher, become more aware that quality matters too.

Finally it made them turn more often to a natural source, versus a packaged one. I am talking vinaigrettes (it really takes only a few minutes to whip a basic yet tasty vinaigrette), homemade chia puddings, fresh vegetables versus canned ones, real organic versus cheaper milk etc.

It is a day to day, conscious decision to be questioning what we put in our mouth. Take a few more minutes at your usual supermarket and decide to study one category of foods that you use as a staple. It could be peanut butter or cereals? Or do you want to study cookies this week?

So today or tomorrow, choose an aisle and a category and analyze labels:

- What is really a serving? How many servings in the package
- How many net carbs are there (Total carbs minus fiber)
- What is this gluten free expensive cookie made of?
- How many net carbs versus protein per serving? Is it respecting a healthy 2 to 1 ratio?
- Why do they say it is sugar free? Is it that they did not add any sugar? Let me read the ingredients list
- Are there cheap fillers? As an example companies add soy protein to peanut butter because it is cheaper than peanuts. Or they add corn cellulose to add fiber but in reality to add cheap bulk.
- Are there trans fats, and if yes, what and how are they listed on the ingredients list
- Remember all the many names sugar can carry in Chapter 2.

Experiment #5: Learn your preservatives

This one is not fun. It will hurt. It will annoy you. It will scare and anger you. Let's become more familiar with the never ending list of preservatives, flavor enhancers, dyes, and additives of all sorts added to or sprinkled on foods, including produce. And then let's just google them.

For instance, what on earth are Butylated Hydroxyanisole (BHA) and Hydroxytoluene (BHT)? Well, they are additives to avoid rancidity and keep colors alive! Yes you do not want your beautiful candies to fade!

What is Sodium Benzoate? Well, it is used to prevent molds from forming in foods, produce and beverages. It can trigger hyperactivity in me and when I arrived in the US, it caused me to develop mouth sores.

Or what is Sodium Nitrite? It is used in processed meats and sausages to preserve them and is linked, in high quantities or when taking chronically, to gastric cancer.

Become an informed eater. Become a critical eater. Become an activist. Question everything. Call companies and complain. Be careful about what you feed your children. Stay vigilant. I feel bad I have to write this. But this is the state of affairs today and with disappearing regulations, including at the environmental level, our soils, water supply and grasses are becoming more polluted. GMO is becoming more difficult to detect and labeling it may become non-mandatory in the U.S.

I am not trying to increase your anxiety level but food nowadays requires all your attention, education and must be taken seriously. We are what we eat. There is no way escaping this truth. It is difficult to be perfect, but we can try to do our best.

There is a source of information that I really like and that I trust: EWG.com or "Know your environment and protect your health." Visit them: www.ewg.org

CogniDiet® Book Club Discussion Guide

This week is focused on your overall health and the attention you pay to it. If you were able to do a pre and post 12 week program blood work with your doctor that would be terrific. It is usually covered by insurances every 3 months. Make sure you ask for:

- **A lipid panel (total cholesterol, HDL, LDL and triglycerides)**
- **Fasting glucose and hemoglobin A1c**
- **You could check your liver enzymes**

If one of you has a glucose monitoring device, it would be interesting to do a test at your meeting before eating and within 2 hours after eating!

- **This is not the last meeting, so focus on what actions you took with your health (self- discovery or making an appointment). What is your priority?**
- **What do you think about The Bredesen Protocol? Are you intrigued? Do you want to give it a try?**
- **Take a few packaged foods and analyze the labels.**
- **Have you decided to start, re-adjust or stop some supplements?**
- **How do you feel in general, you are almost done with the program!**

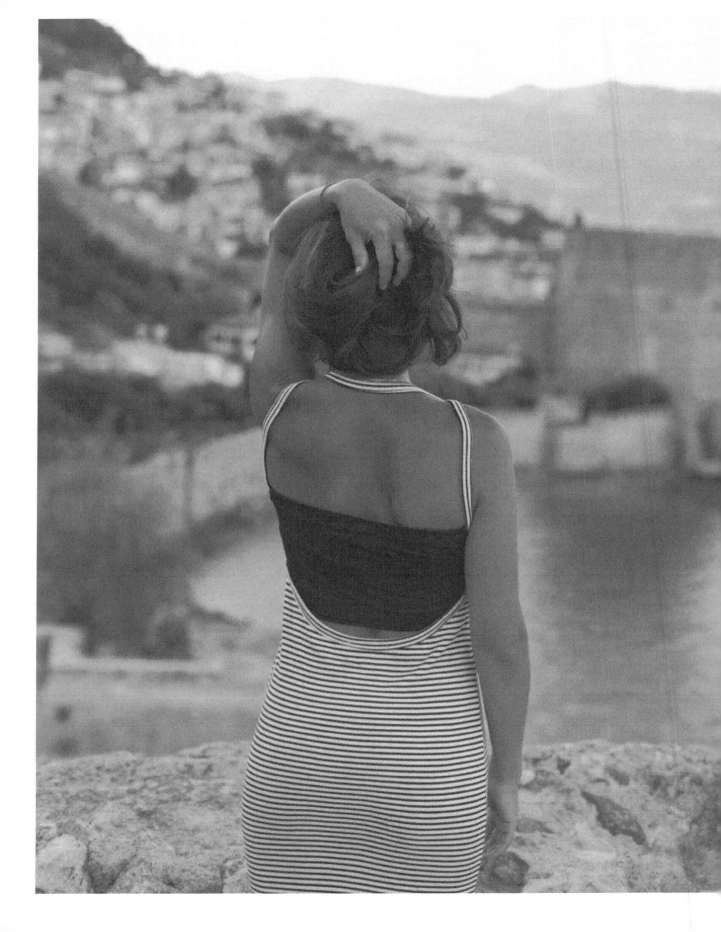

Chapter 12

My Success and My New Goals

This is the end of our time together in this book. I hope we will stay friends. I will continue to support you via my sometimes silly Facebook postings, and all other social media and motivating webinars I am planning. I am already thinking about my next book. It was not as hard as I thought. As I write these lines, I am with you in thoughts. I have gifted my deepest care and creative energy to each word I couched on this paper for you over the past year. This book will help me develop an even better program.

This is only the first part of your self-discovery journey. This is a time to reflect on what has changed within you. This is a time where usually my class participants are amazed, proud, surprised still at their success, and pumped up for the next round. They usually complain about a 12 week program initially; too long, how am I going to do this; this is such a commitment etc. But when the program is over, they just do not want to stop. Hence new curricula, workshops and boot camps to keep the success and motivation going. These have witnessed not only their own blossoming but partners, children or parents may have lost weight as well. There has been a food revolution at home! The confidence level is boosted. Even if the weight loss was minimal, eating habits have changed. Blood work shows amazing improved results.

Jane and Bob's Story

I will always remember a woman, let's call her Jane, who participated in the clinical trial. It is December 2016 and it is the last session. It is crucial for The CogniDiet® to capture this last week's data. This is a serious study. We are in New Jersey and there is a terrible snow storm, compounded with dangerously icy roads. We are expecting the last 7 or 8 participants. I am taking a flight later that day to spend Christmas with my family in Europe. I am panicking. We have to go to plan B. Eventually, most of them will come the next day and my wonderful assistant Joanne will take care of the final weight data collection.

But three local expert drivers still came to the office that day. Jane's husband drove her, how kind. He sat at the meeting table with us. We gave him a coffee. There were the three trial participants and myself. We are all wearing boots and big coats. I remember the participants were worried that their heavy sweaters and pants would sabotage the final weight capture. They stripped down, some of them to their under shirt! We took the time to cover the last session's topics. Jane's husband listened and participated. He was excited. I even convinced him to go on our medical scales and get his body composition done! Now he knew his fat percentage!

This man, let's call him Bob, had started to eat differently at home as well. Jane and Bob were barbecue experts and big steak and potato eaters. They also have a huge family that invaded the house every weekend. They hosted traditional barbecues and welcomed every one. I am talking about 20 people. As per Jane, there were offering mountains of foods.

Jane had lost 27 pounds. She was elated. And her husband had lost pounds during the same 12 weeks. Just by changing the way they cooked at home! No more potato salads and huge juicy burgers, homemade cakes and ice cream gallons. And I am talking huge portions too here. Hello fresh colorful salads, grilled shrimp, roasted chicken and vegetable stews. The potato salad and steak did not disappear completely. But this shows you the power of healthy foods. Jane became very emotional on that day while she was listening to her husband. We were surrounded by a white silence and closed offices. We must have been the only office open in the business park.

I felt the power of love. My love for my clients. Jane's real and genuine appreciation for what we had done for her and her family. Her husband's love too. They braved the storm to help me get the data. A recurring theme was the power of groups and how each participant had supported the others. We had usually 5 to 6 women per class in the trial. But also how deeply personal and soul searching this journey had been as it forced participants to get at the core of what was pushing and driving their former addictions.

I hope you started a "book club" with some of your friends to undertake this journey with The CogniDiet® as I advised earlier. I wish that you enjoyed some of the experiments together with your friends, or your family. Maybe some were implemented with your kids.

Be Proud of Your Achievements

Now is the time to write your achievements, your biggest aha moments and your new goals for the next 6 or 12 months. The results are not officially in yet as I write these lines but I am expecting that 70 to 80% of the trial participants will have continued to lose or maintained their loss 6 months after the end of the trial. 80% was the results for the first cohort, the one that finished in June 2016. They lost another average two pounds after 6 months for a total of 14 pounds. We are analyzing the one year data as I finish this book.

This is what matters the most: enjoying your results. Any result. Even if you are disappointed with your weight results, there are some changes in your habits that are also victories. One participant saw a minimal (her words) weight loss, I am talking 6 pounds, but saw her cholesterol and A1c go seriously down (from 6.5 to 5.8), even after 6 weeks on the program. She changed her eating habits and decided to focus on her weight as her next stage.

Everybody is at a different level of readiness when it comes to weight loss. Some are late bloomers. I had another participant who did not do well. She went up and down 2 to 3 pounds all over the trial. But when she came for her 12 month follow up she had lost 12 more pounds. She said:

"I internalized the information over the past twelve weeks but implemented little change. However, I started to go back to my class binder in January and became more committed. It's as if I had to lose a first layer of resistance in the past 6 months, which I think was my protective gear. I was not ready. Now I have decided to take the second layer off. Losing weight has come easy to me now. I am ready."

So here below please write down, to start with, the list of the habits and behaviors that have changed for you over the past weeks. I believe it is even more important than the weight loss number.

Look at Different Aspects of Your Life	My New Habits or What Has Changed *Start by saying: I….*
Nutrition	Example: I now eat a complete breakfast every morning (Protein/Carb/Fat)
Fitness	Example: I walk three times a week
Stress Reduction	Example: I resigned from this not for profit board that was consuming my energy
Health in General	Example: I have stopped taking antacids as I do not experience gastric reflux anymore

Other: Work, Family, Spirituality, etc.	Example: I take 20 min every evening now to do yoga before I go to bed

How long is the list, how many small and big things have changed? How do you feel in your head and in your soul about yourself now? What have you discovered about yourself? Describe the words, be spontaneous. Free is a word I have heard often. Please don't write anything negative, you have to focus on the positives.

I am feeling (focus on how you feel, not how you are): _____

_____

_____

If you still struggle and have a hard time being positive, here is a trick. You have been able to adopt some new behaviors, even temporarily over the past weeks. Obviously you are trying to change if you got to the end of this book. Each time you did something positive, you created or reinforced a new habit pathway in your brain. So work hard and go back to your journal. And then write the list of each time you experienced a victory. Even, if it is that one time where you refused a dessert. You will be surprised.

Compare Pictures Before and After

Now let's look at your appearance. I advised you to take a picture of yourself (close face and body) before the program. Take these pictures again. What has changed? Besides the weight and the body composition, if you have such scale, what is different?

For example:

- My waist
- My calves, thighs, arms measures
- My face features (cheeks, chin, eyes...)
- My body shape in general
- My clothes sizes
- My energy, mental acuity, fitness stamina, muscle mass, self-confidence, etc.
- My blood numbers or other health indexes. For instance, you do not have to take a blood pressure medication anymore, or can take a lower dose!

Now that you have compiled the list of your successes, please learn to appreciate it and be grateful you received them from the universe.

Cogni-Game:

Once you have written these lists, print them and read them often for a few days. Before you go to bed, close your eyes, appreciate and bask into the pleasure derived from having achieved these goals. Visualize yourself now, versus twelve weeks ago.

Revisit Your Vision Board and Make New Goals

The final exercise today is to go back to your vision board. What has changed? What has been achieved? You had a mountain of vegetables there to inspire you and are now eating like a rabbit. Is this the time to alter the vision board? Maybe there are new goals and aspirations? Some of the vision has been achieved already after a few weeks. One of my client put her new 35 pounds lighter picture in the center of her board, on top of a mountain. In leggings—a novelty for her! She had been able to climb that mountain—OK we are talking about New Jersey. She was not fit enough 12 weeks ago to do it. Her journey consisted of eating well AND getting fit as a priority. She was tired of being a couch potato. Now she belongs to a biking club. And she has lost another

26 pounds.

Include more of your life aspirations in your next board version. After a serious and durable weight loss experience, my clients often start to shift their energy and focus on life in general, whether it is about a new career, going back to school or dumping a couple of energy vampires.

Action: Reflect on your vision board. Changes needed? Goals achieved? New goals in mind?

The decision you took to change has had an impact on your mental and physiological makeover. You are not the same person anymore. It may make some jealous, envious, or happy for you. Some will be inspired. I always ask one thing at the end to my clients. Of course I appreciate testimonials and referrals. But most importantly I want my CogniGirls® to carry on their new spirit and become beacons of joy and positivity.

Sometimes they tell me: "Veronique, it's difficult to really explain what we did with you. It's not really a diet, it's a transformation and people don't get it. They think and hope that there is a secret potion. But I tell them there is no such thing. I am my own secret potion!"

It is time to conclude and thank you again for your confidence. I will just leave you with a summary of my core tenets. They are there for you to remember and stay inspired and committed. At the end it is very simple. My philosophy in life is that we do not have enough time to really count calories every day and measure teaspoons perfectly. We are humans. I hope you noticed that I tried to keep things as simple as possible with the following nutritional priorities:

- Eat fresh as much as you can with at least 5 to 7 cups of vegetables every day
- Eat balanced meals, from breakfast - which is imperative - to dinner
- Link carbohydrates, proteins and fats. Always.
- Remember that glucose is stored as fat if not burned after 20min to 2 hours. And that ALL carbohydrates (except fiber) become glucose in your blood!
- Portions should respect the REASONABLE 11in maximum plate model: ½ veggies- ¼ protein - ¼ starchy carbs max
- Good fat is your friend
- We do not need to eat as much as we think!
- 80% of weight loss is food. You can never outrun your fork!

The core pillars of the CogniDiet® are based on almost 10 years now of helping people and learning what works and what does not work so well. I have met the most motivated dieters and the most resistant participants. But change is possible if you put your heart to it! Here are my 7 truths. These are the principles and learnings I have accumulated over the years:

1. Sugar is sneaky and addictive and will always try to make a comeback.

2. You are a nutrition artist now. Or an expert, whatever label you want to use. You need to continue to work on your talent or your trade. We do not lose weight one day and then move on to another activity. Eating naturally and being attuned to your body needs is your new life style. You are now a constant chiseler.

3. Stress is the biggest saboteur of good health and weight and must be managed. There is no way around that!

4. Exercise is an aging body's best friend. Remember to build these muscles

5. Every change, even the smallest step, is a victory. And yes you can learn to change, even at 74!

6. There is nothing that cannot be achieved if you put your mind to it. The mind precedes the action. The brain pathway to direct and inspire this action must be, and can be built.

7. And finally, have fun, enjoy life, be positive, love yourself, be a little bit crazy (like me), be curious, stay young in your mind. Forget about diet. It has occupied your mind for too long.

The last book club meeting should really focus on discussing your achievements, what has changed and what are your next goals. There is always something new you want to tackle.

Life's routine comes back with full force and I see sometimes my clients feeling alone or lost once the group is over. Maintaining optimal health and weight is really a full time job, let's be honest. But once you have decided, once and for all, where you stand on certain choices, it becomes easy. I, for instance, do not touch pasta anymore. And I do not miss it.

You could decide to continue as a group and become a weekly discussion circle, inviting some experts, cooking and shopping for food together, exercising together, or just continue the contact on your private Facebook page. You could bring your partners in the circle after a while, at least from time to time.

You should be proud of yourselves, create a song, get crazy and dance together, throw a party...I don't know, just have fun and enjoy your life.

Be free, happy and healthy my friend.

With love, Veronique

Bibliography:

Ann Louis Gittleman, M.S., C.N.S. 2002. *Guide to the 40/30/30 Phenomenon*. New York, NY: Contemporary Books, a division of the McGraw-Hill Companies.

Ann Louise Gittleman, M.S., C.N.S. 2003. *Before the Change: Taking Care of Your Perimenopause*. San Francisco, CA: HarperOne, an imprint of HarperCollins Publishers.

Bob Greene. 2006. *The Best Life Diet*. New York, NY: Simon and Schuster

Bob Greene; John J. Merendino Jr., M.D.; Janis Jibrin, M.S., R.D. 2009. *The Best Life Guide to Managing Diabetes and Pre-Diabetes*. New York, NY: Simon and Schuster

Cheryle R. Hart, M.D. and Mary Kay Grossman, R.D. 2007. *The Insulin Resistant Diet*. New York, NY: McGraw-Hill.

Dale Bredesen, M.D., 2017. *The End of Alzheimer's: The First Program to Prevent and Reverse Cognitive Decline*. New York, NY: Penguin Books.

Dallas Hartwig and Melissa Hartwig. *It Starts with Food*. Las Vegas, NV: Victory Belt Publishing.

David M. Nathan, M.D.; Linda M. Delahanty, M.S., R.D. 2005. *Beating Diabetes*. New York, NY: The McGraw-Hill Companies.

David Perlmutter, M.D., with Kristin Loberg. 2016. *The Grain Brain Whole Life Plan: Boost Brain Performance, Lose Weight, and Achieve Optimal Health*. Boston, MA: Little, Brown and Company.

Eliza Kingsford with Debora Yost. 2017. *Brain-Powered Weight Loss*. New York, NY: Rodale Wellness.

Joel Fuhrman, M.D. 2011. Eat to Live: *The Amazing Nutrient-Rich Program for Fast and Sustained Weight Loss*. Boston, MA: Little Brown and Company

Joel Fuhrman, M.D. 2014. *How to Live For Life: The End of Dieting*. San Francisco, CA: HarperOne, an imprint of HarperCollins Publishers.

Jonah Lehrer. 2010. *How We Decide*. New York, NY: First Mariner Books.

Jonathan Haidt. 2006. *The Happiness Hypothesis*. New York, NY: Basics Books of Perseus Books Group.

Judith S. Beck. 1995. *Cognitive Therapy Basics and Beyond*. New York, NY: The Guildford Press.

Judith S. Beck, Ph.D. 2007. *The Beck Diet Solution*. New York, NY: Oxmoor House, an imprint of Time Inc. Books.

Judith S. Beck, Ph.D. 2008. *The Complete Beck Diet for Life*. Birmingham, AL: Oxmoor House, Inc.

Judith Orloff, M.D. 2004. *Positive Energy*. New York, NY: Three Rivers Press, an imprint of the Crown Publishing Group, a division of Random House, Inc.

Judith Orloff, M.D. 2012. *Dr. Judith Orloff's Guide to Intuitive Healing: 5 Steps to Physical, Emotional, and Sexual Wellness*. New York, NY: Random House, LLC.

Laurel Mellin. 2010. *Wired for Joy*. Carlsbad, CA: Hay House, Inc.

Laurel Mellin, M.A, R.D. 2003. *The Pathway*. New York, NY: Harpers Collins Publishers, Inc.

Leslie Beck, R.D. 2001. *The Ultimate Nutrition Guide for Women*. Hoboken, NJ: John Wiley & Sons.

Lucia Capacchione, Ph.D. 2001. *The Art of Emotional Healing*. Boston, MA: Shambhala Publications, Inc.

Michèle Freud. 2003. *Mincir et se réconcilier avec soi*. Paris, France: Editions Albin Michel, S.A.

Michelle May, M.D. 2011. *Eat What You Love, Love What You Eat*. Phoenix, AZ: Am I Hungry? Publishing.

Mark Hyman, M.D. 2014. *The Blood Sugar Solution 10-Day Detox Diet*. New York, NY: Little, Brown and Company, Hachette Book Group.

Mark Hyman, M.D. 2016. *Eat Fat Get Thin*. New York, NY: Little, Brown and Company, Hachette Book Group.

Michael Pollan. 2006. *The Omnivore Dilemma: A Natural History of Four Meals*. New York, NY: Penguin Press.

Michael Pollan. 2013. *Cooked*. New York, NY: Penguin Press.

Miriam E. Nelson, Ph.D. with Sarah Wernick, Ph.D. 1998. *Strong Women Stay Slim*. New York, NY: Bantam Books, a Division of Random House Inc.

Neal D. Barnard, M.D. 2013. *Power Foods for The Brain*. New York, NY: Hachette Book Group.

Richard Shames, M.D., Karilee Shames, Ph.D., R.N. 2005. *Feeling Fat, Fuzzy or Frazzled?* New York, NY: Hudson Street Press, Penguin Group.

Ridha Arem, M.D., 2013. *The Thyroid Solution*. New York, NY: Ballantine Books.

Robert Lustig, M.D., MSL. 2017. *The Hacking of the American Mind: The Science Behind the Corporate Takeover of Our Bodies and Brains*. New York, NY: Penguin Group, LLC.

Roberta L. Duyff, M.S., R.D.N., FAND, CFCS. 2017. *Academy of Nutrition and Dietetics Complete Food & Nutrition Guide (revised edition)*. Boston, MA: Houghton Mifflin Harcourt.

Ruth Q. Wolever, Ph.D. and Beth Reardon, M.S., R.D., L.D.N. with Tania Hanna. 2015. *The Mindful Diet: How to Transform Your Relationship with Food for Lasting Weight Loss and Vibrant Health*. New York, NY: Simon and Schuster.

Shawn Talbott, Ph.D. 2002. *The Cortisol Connection*. Alameda, CA: Hunter House Publishers Inc.

Shawn Talbott, Ph.D. 2004. *The Cortisol Connection Diet*. Alameda, CA: Hunter House Publishers Inc.

Stephen Rollnick, Pip Mason, and Chris Butler. 1999. *Health Behavior Change, a Guide for Practitioners*. London, UK: Churchill Livingstone, an imprint of Elsevier Limited.

Thich Nhat Hanh and Dr. Lilian Cheung. 2010. *Savor, Mindful Eating, Mindful Life*. New York, NY: Harpers Collins Publishers, Inc.

Resources:

The CogniDiet® Resources:

- **Website:** www.thecognidiet.com
- **YouTube:** The CogniDiet https://www.youtube.com/watch?v=Kqu09dzdFpg
- **Facebook:** The Cognidiet - https://www.facebook.com/TheCogniDiet and "The CogniDiet Support Group", a private group for clients only — https://www.facebook.com/groups/1018001928276151/
- **Twitter:** @thecognidiet - https://twitter.com/TheCognidiet
- **Instagram:** @thecognidiet - https://www.instagram.com/thecognidiet/
- **Pinterest:** The CogniDiet - https://www.pinterest.com/thecognidiet/
- **LinkedIn:** Veronique Cardon – https://www.linkedin.com/in/veroniquecardon/
- **LinkedIn:** "The CogniDiet Weight Loss Programs" page — https://www.linkedin.com/company/5309790/

Veronique Cardon, M.S. Interviews:

- Town Topics, Princeton, NJ: http://www.towntopics.com/wordpress/2014/01/08/training-your-brain-to-tame-your-cravings-is-the-target-of-the-cognidiettm-program/

- Suburban Life Magazine, Philadelphia, PA. www.suburbanlifemagazine.com/articles/?articleid=1213

- Podcast with Debbie Lang, The Voice of Real Estate, on Fox Sports Radio 920 The Jersey. Topics as varied as how to make your home healthy for the holidays, how to manage cravings, limit calories and live a healthier life in general. : https://thecognidiet.com/2017/03/debbie-lang-veronique-cardon-talk-tips-make-home-healthier/

Veronique Cardon, M.S. Publications:

CogniDiet Clinical Trial Top Results Abstract /Oral Presentation American College of Nutrition, November 9, 2017:
"COGNIDIET®: A PRELIMINARY STUDY OF THE EFFECTS OF COGNITIVEBEHAVIOR THERAPY AND MINDFULNESS TRAINING ON WEIGHT LOSS AND METABOLIC HEALTH" by Veronique Cardon, MS; Randi Fain, M.D.; Maria Benito, M.D.; Johanna Nordlie, Ph.D.; Pam Kelley, Ph.D." www.tandf.co.uk/journals/pdf/2017_Abstracts_JACN.pdf

Recipe Sites I Like:

- The 100 Best Gluten Free Recipes by Carol Fenster, 2012. Houghton Mifflin Harcourt editions.

- The Suppers Programs Recipes. Full of healthy, plant based and easy to make recipes. They may however sometimes require special spices and ingredients. There are many gluten free recipes. http://www.thesuppersprograms.org/recipes

- Whole 30/Paleo Recipes — http://allrecipes.com/recipes/22590/healthy-recipes/whole30/

- For the rather sophisticated cooks who like aromatics and spices, I love Yotam Ottolenghi books and recipes. https://www.ottolenghi.co.uk/recipes

- Epicurious - For a variety of tips and versatile recipes — https://www.epicurious.com/

- For vegetarians, I recommend to find the most inspiring blogs at http://www.thekitchn.com/eating-vegetarian-5-cooking-blogs-to-check-out-now-188840

- There are a few of my recipes on my own website, just go to the recipe section: https://thecognidiet.com/category/recipes/

Stress relief:

If you don't have time to take a bath or a massage, you can use a few apps.

- The Pacifica app (stress and anxiety using CBT and mindfulness) — https://itunes.apple.com/us/app/pacifica-for-stress-anxiety/id922968861?mt=8

- Hear and Now to learn how to breathe. Will take your stress level with your finger on the phone! https://itunes.apple.com/us/app/hear-and-now-breathe-for-stress-anxiety-relief/id977650202?mt=8

- Coloring books on line with Colorify — http://www.colorfy.net/

About the Author

Veronique Cardon, M.S., is a Holistic Nutritionist with a Master's degree (summa cum laude) in Holistic Nutrition from the Clayton College of Natural Health. She started to meditate in 2005 and gained a Certificate of Completion in Cognitive Behavioral Therapy (CBT) applied to weight loss at The Beck Institute for the Advancement of Human Behavior in July 2013. She also holds a Commercial Engineer degree (magna cum laude) from the University of Brussels, Belgium. She led a successful career in the pharmaceutical industry in the U.S. and Europe and attended special management and leadership programs at INSEAD in France and the Harvard Business School in the U.S. She serves on the board of trustees of The Suppers Programs, a non-profit organization based in Princeton, NJ, whose mission is to help people lead healthier lives by eating deliciously prepared whole foods in a supportive setting.

About the Consulting Editors

Clifford N. Lazarus, Ph.D., is a licensed psychologist and Director of The Lazarus Institute (TLI). In addition to his Multimodal CBT psychotherapy practice, he specializes in neuropsychology and collaborative psychopharmacology. He received his BA, MS, and Ph.D. in psychology from Rutgers University where he was a Henry Rutgers Research Scholar. Since 2000, Dr. Lazarus has been a consultant for Global Medical Institutes (Formerly Princeton Biomedical Research), a leading facility dedicated to the highest standards of research integrity in evaluating new generation medications. He is the current, world authority on Multimodal Therapy as originated by his late father, Professor Arnold A. Lazarus, Ph.D., ABPP. Dr. Lazarus has authored numerous professional publications and books. He is also the author of a widely used therapy assessment questionnaire, the "Multimodal Life-History Inventory." He is a regularly featured blogger for "Psychology Today" for which he has authored many dozens of blog posts. Read more at http://thelazarusinstitute.com/

Shelley Weinstock, Ph.D., CNS, FACN, is a nutritional biochemist, researcher, teacher and clinician. She earned her BA in Chemistry from Bard College and her Ph.D. in Nutritional Biochemistry from the Massachusetts Institute of Technology. After a Post-Doctoral fellowship at Harvard School of Public Health, she focused on teaching and basic research in the nutrition-related diseases at Barnard College and Montclair University. She has worked in the nutraceutical industry and consulted with pharmaceutical companies. Dr. Weinstock currently teaches and advises students at the Institute of Human Nutrition at Columbia University Medical Center, has a private nutrition practice in NJ and consults for start-ups, academia and non-profits. Read more at: www.weinstocknutrition.com

Acknowledgements

I want to first of all thank all my clients for their support, confidence and inspiration. Their stories are in this book. I will never forget Sharon, my first client ever. I framed her first check! And four years later, at 65, she is still 40 pounds lighter!

Thank you to Clifford Lazarus, Ph.D. and Shelley Weinstock Ph.D., CNS, for their insights, scientific feedback and expertise in cognitive behavior therapy, and in nutrition respectively. They also added the value of their large experience with their own patients to this book.

Maria Benito, M.D., and Randi Fain, M.D. for their friendship, expertise, support, and medical input in the development and implementation of our clinical trial in 2016. Rick Weiss, Ph.D. gave me a break when I purchased his Viocare® nutritional assessment tool for the trial and was always ready to share a cup of coffee in Princeton, NJ, to advise me on my trial and more.

Karen Hodges Miller, from Open Door Publications, for her candid and honest editing. Many times she had to reel me back into the real world of women, outside the corporate lingo I had lived with for so long. Plus, she discovered a few words and phrases than only a French girl would write! She also encouraged me many times when the writer's emotional block had gotten me in its grip.

Johanna Nordlie, Ph.D., co-author on my first abstract accepted at the American College of Nutrition 58th meeting as an oral presentation in November 2017. Without her there would be no abstract!

Eric Labacz, my wonderful designer. He had to work with so many boxes and Cogni-Tips but managed to create a nice and clear layout for this book.

Joanne, my patient assistant, who has supported me in the most effective way, taking the day to day work-related issues off of my back. She also did some research for me.

My very good friend Delphine. For many years she has listened to my ideas and projects, did some planning with me, offered free advice, found experts, gave constructive criticism and most importantly encouraged me.

Finally I want to thank my family. My daughters Camille and Pauline. How many times did they edit some of my other publications, especially Camille. They also helped me understand social media and the appropriateness (or not) of a post on Instagram®. My loving and soooo patient husband Paul who cooked for me and took care of me every day of this year long journey. His wife was gone, on her computer, in the TV room, most of the time in 2017. I stopped all social life and dedicated every free hour to this book. My sister Muriel who was my first reader and advised me to be less scientific (hope I succeeded) and bring more humor into this book.

Clients and clinical trial participants

Vickie McC., 55 years old, is 25 pounds lighter, still one year after the trial. "This is not a diet, this is freedom. I have been on diets for 50 years, with very short lasting effects. I am enjoying life in a way I didn't know was possible. Imagine a day that you don't wake up thinking about what you are going to eat!"

Cheryl R., 51 years old, is 30 pounds lighter, still one year after the trial. "The CogniDiet® has changed my life. It is not a diet but an education in changes in food behavior and nutrition! I've lost 30 pounds without depriving myself, became a mindful eater by making good choices and I am more active and physically stronger."

Lynne R., 70 years old, is 36 pounds lighter, still 18 months after the trial: "Veronique's guidance was invaluable. It has made me much more aware of what I eat. It taught me to think about food and my overall health in a more complete way. The CogniDiet® Program gave me a more realistic attitude about what it means to be successfully in control of my eating."

Deb S., 57 years old and a vegetarian, is 39 pounds lighter, still 6 months after the trial: "I feel like a big burden has been taken away from my shoulders. A feeling of helplessness. A sense I could never win this war with sugar. Little did I know how badly I was eating. Yet, it was so simple to change."

Made in the USA
Middletown, DE
20 March 2019